WOMEN WARRIORS IN INDIAN HISTORY

Yugal Joshi grew up in a remote village of Uttarakhand, and has walked across diverse territories while working in government, public and private sectors.

An alumnus of IIT Delhi and NUS Singapore, he is the co-author of authoritative books on Singapore's water management, *The Singapore Water Story*, and on sustainable development, *Creating Shared Values*. He has also authored the novel *Ram: The Soul of Time*.

A keen student of history and a water enthusiast, he is currently Director, Swachh Bharat Mission, and lives in New Delhi with his wife and two children.

WOMEN WARRIORS IN INDIAN HISTORY

YUGAL JOSHI

RUPA

Published by
Rupa Publications India Pvt. Ltd 2017
7/16, Ansari Road, Daryaganj
New Delhi 110002

Sales Centres:

Allahabad Bengaluru Chennai
Hyderabad Jaipur Kathmandu
Kolkata Mumbai

This is a work of fiction. All situations, incidents, dialogue and characters, with the exception of some well-known historical and public figures mentioned in this novel, are products of the author's imagination and are not to be construed as real. They are not intended to depict actual events or people or to change the entirely fictional nature of the work. In all other respects, any resemblance to persons living or dead is entirely coincidental.

ISBN: 978-81-291-4522-2

First impression 2017

10 9 8 7 6 5 4 3 2 1

Printed by

In memory of my elder brother,
Dr Lalit Mohan Joshi,
who introduced me to the joy of reading.

Contents

Author's Note

Finding women warriors in world history is a difficult exercise, and India is no exception. Valour was seldom associated with women in ancient India and found no mention in classical Sanskrit literature. Therefore, obviously when Shridhardas put together his grand compilation of 2,380 Sanskrit poems of about 500 poets in 1205–06 AD, he could not find a single poem even remotely connecting women with valour. It is hardly a surprise that in Goddess Durga's country, the first well chronicled warrior woman in Indian history appears only in the thirteenth century, a few decades after the publication of Shridhardas's compilation.

The choice of warriors in this book is personal and I have not included any lady of recent times, though there are many worthy of mention.

The stories are put together chronologically to cover a large period of Indian history, beginning from the Slave Dynasty to the First War of Indian Independence. Each chapter brings an echo of its times and the reader may see history unfolding before her eyes. An underlying continuity between the chapters ensures that the reader senses the most turbulent six hundred years of Indian history from the perspective of women of the ruling class.

A unique way of storytelling has been used in exploring the life and times of ten Indian women warriors in present book, *Women Warriors in Indian History.* Barring Tara Bai's story, where she herself is the narrator, famous historical characters who were close contemporaries of these heroines narrate the stories. This fictitious intrusion of the narrators sets the role of these warriors in historical perspective, and highlights the issues of their times, for a better understanding of their actions. The narrators—Emperor Jahangir, eunuch General Malik Kafur, legendary Tara Bai, Tatya Tope and Lakshmi Bai, travellers Marco Polo and Pietro Della Valle, writer John Lang and Mary Palmer, wife of Philip Taylor—the author of *Confessions of a Thug*, enrich the book in content and curiosity.

All these warrior women were princesses, queens or regents. Their commitment to cause not only dwarfed the stature of their contemporary male counterparts but also emphasized the freshness of ideas introduced by them in governance. The stories are not merely tales of their bravery in the battlefield, but are curiously blended with socio-political and religious milieu for a better understanding of their personality.

Covering over 600 years of Indian history, the stories are well researched and presented in a lucid and conversational style, with a dash of fiction. The stories will mesmerize the readers with highs and lows of these magnificent characters, and vivid scenes of their exceptional lives.

Yugal Joshi
Ram Navami, 2073
15 April 2016

Raziya Sultan

On a pleasant morning, Malik Kafur, the regent, was telling stories of the late sultan—Ala-ud-din Khalji—to his pupil and present sultan, Malik Shihab-ud-din. They were sitting in a balcony of the Siri Fort, also known as the 'Palace of Thousand Pillars' in Dilli. After a ruthless winter, the weather had become pleasant.

The young Sultan was only six years old and Malik Kafur, the confidant and chief advisor of Ala-ud-din for last fifteen years, held the real power. The grand political edifice of the compulsive workaholic, Ala-ud-din Khalji was built upon Malik Kafur's stunning victories over Devagiri, Chittor, Warangal, Hoysala and Madurai, which produced countless wealth.

Malik Kafur was an extraordinary person. A eunuch slave, captured by Ala-ud-din's army at Khambhat, he was called Hazar Dinari, for the exorbitant prize paid by his first owner. An Islamized Hindu, Malik Kafur's beauty captivated Ala-ud-din so much that from the first day of their meeting they became intimate associates.

After the death of Crown Prince Khijr Khan and the imprisonment of powerful Khalji amirs, the highly ambitious

Malik Kafur wanted to rule Hindustan through a puppet sultan. Shihab was his best bet and he took upon himself to teach Shihab the history and administration. Praising Ala-ud-din's administrative reforms, Kafur rated him as one of the finest administrators of the world.

'Why do you call Abba the most extraordinary ruler in the world history?'

'The Sultan was a radical reformer. Whatever he touched turned into gold. More than us, the coming generations will appreciate his work. He was ahead of his time.'

'But, Barani tells me that Abba had prohibited Hindus from riding horses, carrying weapons, wearing fine cloths and chewing betel leaf...'

'What Barani says is correct.'

Malik Kafur, did not show any remorse to a young Shihab, son of Ala-ud-din's Rajput wife, Kamala Devi.

'Shihab, it is out of fear of the late Sultan that no Hindu raises his head. You won't find a sign of gold, silver or any article of luxury in their houses. They are in such an impoverished state that their wives now work in the houses of the Mussulmans for their livelihood.'

A stunned Shihab looked at his mentor for long and then asked in a low voice.

'Malik Naib, has it been like this since the Sultanate was established?'

The question made Malik pause. He was a straightforward man, a brilliant military commander, though quite unskilled in manipulative politics. The image of Raziya flashed before his eyes, as did his long cherished dream—*if a woman can rule from Delhi, why cannot a great warrior eunuch?*

'No Shihab, it was not always like this. There was once a female ruler in Delhi—Raziya Sultan. She defied all the rules of the patriarchal society and ruled the kingdom from her seat. Raziya and her father Iltutmish were the only two sultans who were tolerant towards kafirs. Raziya, in fact, abolished jajia during her reign. If she had ruled longer, she would have been a great queen. Pity, she only got three turbulent years at the helm.'

The young Sultan was intrigued to hear about the Queen. 'Please tell me about her,' young Shihab requested Malik.

'Shihab, I know no other woman in the Mussulman society, who had ever sat on the throne. Despite the purdah restrictions, Raziya ruled the empire with distinction. She was endowed with all the qualities befitting a king. But, she was not born in the right sex…' said Malik Kafur, and his thoughts turned to his situation.

'*Why do men think only they can rule, why can't the women?*'

He bit his lower lip.

'*One day, I will rule Hindustan.*'

'Then?' unaware of Kafur's reverie, an innocent Shihab asked.

'As she was a woman who dared to rule like a man, she was overthrown in three years and killed by a band of orthodox amirs.'

'But why would they do that? Tell me everything about her,' Shihab urged.

'Shihab, since ages the migrant invaders chose Hindustan as a traget because of its reputation for fabulous riches. Hindustan was considered a soft state, primarily because Turkish cavalry was far superior to the native cavalry in every respect, in men as well as in mounts. Hindi elephant corps were no match to the storming, whirling charge of the Turkish cavalry. In the early eighth century, the first Arab army invading Sindh was commanded by a seventeen year old lad, Muhammad Qasim.' Kafur began the fascinating tale of the Slave Dynasty.

'For three centuries, the Arabs ruled Sindh, but all through its history, the Arab rule remained of little significance in Hind's history.'

'Hindu rulers must have ended their rule then?' Shihab guessed.

'No.' Kafur laughed. 'Hindu rulers were accustomed to live a sedentary life and their armies were always defensive. They still suffer from a victim's syndrome. Arabs and Turks never suffered military reverses in Hind, except in Tarain in 1191.

'The Arab kingdom was wiped out by another Mussulman invader, Mahmud Ghazni, a Turk. Mahmud led more than a dozen campaigns into Hindustan and always returned victorious. But, he had no hunger for the land. He just wanted to gather plunder and slaughter heathens.'

'Then who had established the Sultanate in Hind?' Shiahb asked.

'The Sultanate at Dilli was established by Qutb-ud-din Aibak, the founder of the Slave Dynasty in 1206. It was called the Slave Dynasty because Aibak was a slave of Muhammad Ghuri, who decisively won Hind and began an entirely new epoch in Hind's history. The Slave Dynasty ruled the Sultanate for eighty-four years.

'Aibak's sudden death stirred a debate surrounding succession. The amirs preferred Iltutmish, a meritorious slave and an able officer, to the sons of Aibak. Iltutmish was a Turk of Ilbari tribe and was sold into slavery by his envious brothers as a child. Aibak bought him for one lakh chital coins and never repented. The boy's rank and honour increased steadily and soon he became the chief huntsman. Aibak also made him his son-in-law. Raziya was the daughter of Qutb Begum and Iltutmish.

'How can a slave rule the Sultanate?' the novice Sultan quizzed.

'Shihab, sultans of the Slave Dynasty were all manumitted slaves or their descendants. They were not however ordinary slaves, but royal slaves, and they, far from being an underclass, constituted a privileged politico-military aristocracy, who could aspire for the highest offices in the Sultanate.' Kafur explained.

'Iltutmish ascended the throne in troubled times. The western frontier was unsafe; Yildiz was creating trouble in Ghazni; a rebellion was brewing in Afghan mountains; Qabacha had revolted in Lahore; the Mongols under Genghis Khan were fast approaching the Sindhu River; and Ali Mardan had declared himself independent in Bengal. After Aibak's death, several of the Hindu rajas broke free from the control of the Sultanate and became aggressive.

'Iltutmish was able to overcome most of the problems he faced and established his authority on land which stretched from Ghazni to Bengal. He managed to keep the stormy Turkish amirs under his command and maintained strict discipline in the court. He was just, pious and virtuous. His benevolent reign resulted in the loss of status for the powerful amirs. As a reaction, the amirs formed an informal league called The Forties to counter the supremacy of the Sultan.'

'But where is Raziya? Tell me about Raziya,' young Shihab was getting impatient.

'Without knowing Iltutmish, how can you appreciate Raziya's story, Sultan?'

Shihab nodded his head in agreement, and became quite to allow Kafur with the story.

Iltutmish and Qutb Begum had four sons and two daughters. The eldest son and the crown prince was Nasir-ud-din Mahmud, followed by Gayas-ud-din, Muizz-ud-din and Qutb-ud-din. Raziya and Saziya were the two daughters. But Qutb Begum was not the only wife of Iltutmish. He had many high-born wives and one low-born wife, Shah Turkan, who was his former handmaid. Shah Turkan was a petty, vindictive and vicious woman with very high ambitions. She wanted to rule Delhi through her son Rukn-ud-din, who spent his time indulging in excessive luxuries and enjoyment. A frustrated Iltutmish appointed him the Subedar* of Badayun, hoping that the burden of responsibility might cure him from his addictions. But that never happened. Over the period, especially after the death of Qutb Begum, Shah Turkan and her son Rukn-ud-din became very powerful and evil.

Qutb Begum's death had raised many eyebrows; Nasir-ud-din and Raziya suspected Shah Turkan's hand behind it. But the late queen's body bore no marks of injury or foul play. Lack of evidence forced Raziya to not pursue the matter.

After the death of Qutb Begum, the palace came under

*A subedar is the governor of a province.

the complete influence of Shah Turkan, and Raziya and her siblings were isolated. Things became worse when the crown prince Nasir was sent to Bengal as subedar. The path now lay uncontested for Shah Turkan and Rukn-ud-din and to plot conspiracies against the others.

As the wheel of conspiracies spun faster in the palace, an assassination attempt was made on the Sultan. During a Friday prayer, when the Sultan was offering prayers at the Great Mosque in Dilli, a band of Ismailis stormed inside the prayer hall and cut through the congregation and advanced towards the Sultan. An Abyssinian slave', Jalal ud din Yaqut's quick actions saved the Sultan, who could barely manage to escape before the paid assassins reached him.

Soon after, Raziya received the worst news from Bengal—the eldest and favourite son of Iltutmish, Nasir had died under mysterious circumstances. This misfortune devastated the Sultan. A few months later, while Iltutmish was steering a campaign against the wild Khokars in Punjab, he fell grievously ill and had to return to Dilli.

Raziya's affection towards Yaqut deepened when he saved the life of her father from the Ismilis. But this affinity with the Abyssinian slave became the talk of the town while Shah Turkan and her men fanned the rumours. The spectacular rise of Yaqut to the high offices of the Sultanate was deeply resented by Shah Turkan. She made several attempts to end Raziya's life. One afternoon, Raziya was riding her horse on the bank of River Jamuna when someone shot a poisonous arrow at her. Fortunately, the assassin missed his target and was arrested by Yaqut. However, before the assassin could reveal anything, he consumed poison and died.

When all her attempts came to a naught, Shah Turkan discussed the succession issue with her advisor.

'How do I make Rukn-ud-din the next Sultan? This worry won't let me sleep and is driving me insane.'

'Begum, there is a way.'

'What's that?'

'Vizier Zaidi...'

Vizier Zaidi was famous for his greed. But he had always followed the dictates of the Sultan. He had a great influence over other amirs but was considered a bit timid unless offered a great temptation.

'No. He is very shrewd. I had tried earlier too, but failed. We cannot trust him.'

Despite her hesitation, Shah Turkan decided to take help from Zaidi and as a bribe for supporting Rukn-ud-din, offered valuable gems and the post of Vizier-e-Azam to old Zaidi. Old Zaidi agreed to help her, albeit discretely.

The Sultan's health was slowly declining when one day, the amirs of The Forties, under the leadership of Vizier Zaidi and Sheikh-ul-Islam, urged Iltutmish to nominate a successor.'

'Can amirs do that?' Shihab was surprised.

'Not in the Khalji Sultanate.' Malik Kafur explained. 'The Sultanate during its early years was bedevilled by internecine rivalries and conflicts. The stature of the sultan was that of a first among equals than that of a sovereign like now. In such a situation, you can imagine the pull and push between the sultan and the amirs for sharing power. The amirs always tried to be the masters of their master. During times of royal succession, the amirs invariably tried to test the mettle of the new sultan and always tried to put their own puppet on the royal seat.'

Kafur paused for a while and continued, 'That's why, the amirs went to the dying Sultan and appealed.

'Sultan, we urge you to nominate a successor.' Sheikh, an influential amir, pleaded. 'Sultan, this is the only way to avert the horrors of a disputed succession.'

'I nominate Raziya as my successor,' the Sultan announced, without blinking an eye.

Suddenly, the court was plunged in silence. After a few seconds, Zaidi found his voice.

'May I know on what grounds does the Sultan nominate Raziya?'

Sultan looked into the eyes of old Zaidi and announced again. 'Vizier, I am firm on my decision. She is a distinguished administrator, a brave warrior and a visionary leader. She remains undeterred even in the face of adversity. These are the qualities of a just and ideal Sultan.'

'What about Rukn-ud-din?' asked Zaidi hesitatingly and then added, 'Or your other sons?'

'My sons are devoted to the pleasures of youth, and not one of them is qualified to be the sultan.'

'Rukn-ud-din is doing reasonably well in Badayun,' Zaidi argued.

"Reasonably well' is not good enough to rule Hindustan,' thundered Iltutmish. 'Sahiban, the choice of Raziya is not a sentimental one. I have given a lot of thought to it. She has good administrative skills and whenever I have been away from Dilli, she has carried out the royal duties with great dignity.'

'Sultan, how can we defy conventions?' Balban argued.

'Balban, since when have conventions taken precedence over the welfare of people?'

'But, Raziya is a woman,' said Malik Salari, finally conveying the opinion of The Forties.

'Amirs, after my death you will find that there is no one more competent to guide the state than my daughter.'

The crestfallen courtiers walked out. Iltutmish called his personal assistants and wrote a will. He recorded Raziya's name as his heir.

In the evening, many amirs met Shah Turkan. 'Respected amirs, a royal woman, however ambitious and able she may be, can devise politics only from behind the harem veil, and not openly,' she said.

'I abhor the idea of being subservient to a woman,' Vizier Zaidi announced his sentiment.

'That night, Sultan Iltutmish passed away. Raziya spent the whole night sitting close to her father's side. Disregarding the late king's choice, the amirs placed Rukn-ud-din on the throne. Shah Turkan and Vizier Zaidi quickly completed the proceedings. Only Qutb-ud-din, the youngest son of Iltutmish, protested. For that, he was promptly imprisoned. The final procession of the late Sultan could only start after the new Sultan was coronated.

'Within a few days, the amirs realized that in reality, they were all under the rule of a woman—Shah Turkan. Rukn-ud-din had no interest in ruling and he left all the power to his mother.

'He is entirely feckless,' a frustrated amir, Altunia protested.

'But, he is generous,' said Vizier-e-Azam Zaidi in support of the Sultan.

'His generosity will make us all beggars,' Malik Salari said angrily.

'Rukn-ud-din is so generous and handsome,' said Zaidi, 'no king in any reign has ever distributed gifts, robes of honour and grants the way he does.'

Altunia protested vehemently, 'Vizier-e-Azam, this generosity is a garb to cover his vices.' He looked at the other amirs at the gathering, who were nodding their head in support. 'He is addicted to revelry and debauchery, and bestows his honours and rewards on the bands of singers, buffoons and catamites.'

'Yesterday, he was riding out drunk on an elephant through the bazaars of Dilli, throwing tankas of red gold. People were picking up the coins and rejoicing,' Malik Aitigin said.

'Vizier,' Salari said, 'we cannot bear his inordinate addiction to pleasure and misplaced conviviality.'

'We don't have options. Give him three more months.' Zaidi concluded the meeting of The Forties.

Meanwhile, to establish her complete control in the royal household, Shah Turkan started liquidating her opponents and their supporters. Her blind fury and vindictiveness made life very difficult in the harem. She set about avenging the indignities that she had suffered earlier, and subjected all the wives of Iltutmish to ignominious deaths. She once again hatched a plot to kill Raziya, but failed.

'I cannot suffer these fools,' Malik Salari, now the Subedar of Badayun wrote to Gayas-ud-din, the second son of Iltutmish and the Subedar of Awadh.

'In this environment of gross misrule, it is our divine duty to fight against these two satans,' Gayas-ud-din wrote back to all the provincial governors. Awadh was in the middle of a Sultanate that stretched from Multan to Bengal. Gayas-ud-din's purposeful provocation and high handedness of Rukn-ud-din and Shah Turkan mobilized the provincial governors.

'In rebellion, Gayas-ud-din looted the royal treasure bearers passing through his area. In retaliation, Shah Turkan first blinded Qutb-ud-din and later put him to death.

'To suppress the provincial rebellion, Rukn-ud-din marched out. Meanwhile, the shrewd Vizier-e-Azam, Zaidi joined the rebels and escaped from Dilli to Badayun.

'Once Rukn-ud-din left Dilli, Raziya finally got her chance. She came out from her chamber in a red outfit.

'Why red?' her servant Gul-e-Abbasi asked.

'Red is the colour for a petitioner. I am seeking justice in the court of people. I have the nomination document from the late Sultan, who had chosen me as his successor in presence of legal witnesses. I also have the royal seal.'

'But, the Sultan...'

'Gul, the royal treasure belongs to awam, but the Sultan is spending it mindlessly on jokers and magicians. My brothers and relatives have been killed without reason and Shah Turkan has made many attempts on my life. Today, I shall seek justice from the people of Dilli.'

'Raziya reached the grand mosque where thousands of people had assembled. She was riding a white horse and the people made way for her while respectfully bowing their heads. Public sentiment was overwhelmingly in her favour; Raziya incited a popular uprising.

'Are you happy with the present regime?' she asked the crowd.

'No!' the crowd shouted in one voice, so loud that Rukn-ud-din was said to have heard it near Panipat.

'Who should be your ruler?'

'Raziya, Raziya...,' the people began to chant.

'My awam is my conscience keeper and the real ruler. If someone has any doubts please come forward,' she said.

'Once you become our ruler, what would be your first priority?' someone asked aloud. The crowd went silent in breathless anticipation.

'My first priority is the peace and happiness of people of our kingdom.'

'How would you deal with Rukn-ud-din and Shah Turkan?' a loud voice asked.

'They deserve death,' many in the crowd shouted.

'No one would get punishment without a proper trial. If only they're proved guilty, they will be punished,' Raziya replied.

'Would you give equal rights to Ismaili Shiyas?' someone from the front row asked. The crowd again fell silent. Everyone knew how a gang of Ismailis had tried to assassinate her father.

'Why only Ismailis? In my rule, every citizen will have equal rights.'

'Is it true for women also?'

'Allah, the most benevolent and creator of all, does not distinguish between the two, then why should we?' Raziya's reply stunned the assembly.

Then, an old man came forward and asked in a loud voice, 'Now, you the people, do you accept Raziya as your ruler?'

A chorus of 'Yes! Yes!' filled the sky.

'My awam, it was I whom Abba Huzur had chosen as his successor. But, someone else usurped the crown against the late Sultan's commands. That is the reason for your misery. If

I am better than any man, you may keep me on the throne. If you think otherwise, you may remove the crown from my head and give it to whomsoever you please.'

'The crowd clapped and formed a huge procession to the fort, on its way back. The amirs did not dare go against the popular sentiment and consoled each other saying, 'A daughter is better than an ill-bred son.'

'Thus, on a sunny afternoon in November 1236, Raziya was pronounced the Sultan by public demand and she went on to assume the title, 'Raziya-ud-din', and issued coins in her name. Shah Turkan was arrested and imprisoned. On his return, Rukn-ud-din was also arrested and later killed.'

Shihab was stunned by the story. He didn't utter a word, and heard Kafur with rapt attention. Kafur smiled looking at Shihab so engrossed in the story.

'Shihab, it was the only instance in history when the Hindi awam chose their ruler.' Malik told his protégé. 'Sultan, Raziya always enjoyed tremendous public support and that was the reason why, despite many efforts of The Forties, every attempt to dethrone her failed.'

Raziya's accession was also resented by the subedars. The former Vizier, Zaidi, encouraged provincial subedars to dethrone Raziya. A combined force of Malik Jani, Malik Kuchi, Malik Kabir Khan and Malik Salari converged outside Dilli. In response, Raziya took her camp outside Dilli, to the banks of River Jamuna and with her clever diplomacy, sowed dissension among the amirs. Salari and Kabir Khan covertly joined Raziya and as a result, the confederacy scattered and the fleeing rebels were chased and captured. Kuchi and his brother were captured and killed. Amir Zaidi fled to the Sirmur hills and died there. Raziya's swift action earned her the admiration of many amirs, and won them over to her side. Rebellion was extinguished from Deval to Lakhnauti.

Once all chords of the kingdom came into her hands, Raziya broke free from the traditional restrictions laid on the harem ladies. She sat in the open court and took all major decisions of the Sultanate herself. With every passing day, she became bolder in her conduct in royal court and made regular public appearances.

The orthodox umra and influential amirs in The Forties sulked but could not oppose her actions openly. They waited for an excuse or an opportune moment to strike back.

After three years had passed, Raziya threw off the dress and veil that the women wore and put on a tunic and cap, and appeared in public riding a horse like men do—armed with a bow and quiver, and surrounded by the courtiers.

'Look, she has no veil on her face,' Kabir Khan said.

'What else do you expect?' Aitigin said, disgustedly. 'Among all the men in this world, she could find that Abyssinian Yaqut for companionship and intimacy. How can we accept this amorous relationship?'

'You are Amir-i-Hazib and that slave is Amir-i-Akhur! Now, the Abyssinians will teach us how to manage our stables,' said Altunia.

'She likes strong fellows, Altunia,' Aitigin hit back.

'More than her yearning for intimacy with that slave, have you noticed how she is reducing the power of The Forties?' Kabir Khan questioned.

'How?'

'All these high offices are traditionally run by the Turk amirs. Now, she is appointing slaves and the Indian Mussulmans to the high offices, thus reducing our influence. I am already shunted out to Lahore,' Kabir Khan explained.

After a few days of this incident, Kabir Khan revolted. Raziya took no time to suppress the rebellion and removed Kabir Khan from the subedari of Lahore.

'We cannot win her through our individual efforts,' Aitigin declared in a meeting of The Forties.

'She cannot be ousted in Dilli. The people will not allow us to do so.' Altunia's logic was sound.

'I agree. Let us join hands and drag her out of Dilli,' said Aitigin, and hatched a conspiracy to depose Raziya.

Problems for Raziya were increasing. Her brother Gayas-ud-din died under suspicious circumstances and the resenting amirs were vilifying her in public for her suspected amorous relationship with Yaqut. She sensed the rebels' plan and reshuffled her office holders to appease the prominent amirs. Amir-i-Hazib Aitgin was also made the Subedar of Badayun and Altunia was given charge of a bigger province, Tabarhind.

Despite the attempt for appeasement, The Forties continued hatching conspiracies.

'Let us place Prince Muiz-ud-din on the throne. He is young and inexperienced, so I will be his deputy,' Aitigin moved his small eyes.

'I don't care. Yaqut should be killed. I want my province, the post of Vizier and Raziya,' Altunia agreed.

'I promise, one day you will marry her,' Aitigin assured Altunia.

Altunia rebelled in Tabarhind. Raziya, in the sweltering heat of the summer of 1240, moved out of Dilli to quell the rebellion. The rebels swung into full action and many close associates of Raziya, including Yaqut, were killed. Razia was arrested and imprisoned in Bhatinda Fort.

Aitigin fulfilled his promise and handed over Raziya to his accomplice.

'Then?' An apprehensive Shihab interrupted Kafur.

'Shihab, remember Raziya was only down, not out.' Kafur thought to tell Shihab about Altunia.

'Sultan, you see, since his youth, Altunia had nursed a desire to marry Raziya. Now, she was his captive. Tender feelings towards Raziya restricted him to take any drastic action against her. Raziya knew it very well and decided to use the lure of high office and her company to entice Altunia, to ally with her.

When Altunia visited her, she decided to agree to marry him.'

'Malik, please don't address me as sultan. I am your prisoner,' she said.

'Sultan, pardon me. Not you, but I am your prisoner. Please forgive me for this inconvenience,' Altunia apologized, overcome with emotion.

'Raziya, you have been in my heart for years.'

'I know that,' Raziya smiled. 'I am ready to marry you, but I have a few conditions.'

'Anything, Sultan,' Altunia consented.

'Let our marriage be simple.'

'Only that? Done.'

'No, one more. Promise me that you will continue our fight against the rebels until you sit on the throne of Hindustan.

'I accept all your conditions,' Altunia bowed his head.

The next day, Raziya married Altunia. Together, they advanced to Dilli with an army of twenty thousand.

In Dilli, Aitigin's tenure as Naib-i-Mamlikat was short lived. His expectations to use Sultan Muiz-ud-din Baharam Shah as a puppet could not be fulfilled. As an individual Baharam Shah was a bizarrely inconsistent and whimsical person. From the day he sat on the throne, the Sultan looked upon Aitigin with great suspicion. The Sultan was always wary of his scheming minister.

One day, when the Sultan passed by Aitigin's mansion, he saw an elephant and a military music band at its entrance, a practice that was allowed only at the royal palace. An angry Baharam Shah promptly executed Aitigin.

Baharam Shah sent a huge force to counter Raziya and Altunia. Outside of Dilli, Raziya's fortune had never backed her; in the ensuing battle, her army was completely defeated by Bahram Shah's forces.

'Not even a horseman is with us,' a worried Altunia looked around.

Together, they fled from the battlefield. She asked for shelter from the residents of Kaithal but once she entered the premises, the locals imprisoned her.

Raziya and Altunia were killed in Kaithal. Everyone knew of her love for Dilli and she was buried on the banks of River

Jamuna where a small tomb was erected to mark her grave.

Kafur became silent. He looked at the young Sultan and then said in a soft voice, 'Sultan, can you see that small tomb in the Turkman area? That is Raziya's tomb. It has now become a pious place.'

Malik Kafur took a deep breath and then completed his story, 'Shihab, Sultan Raziya was a great monarch. She had all the qualities of a great king. But, she was not of the *right* sex.'*

*Keay, J. (2000) *India*, Harper Press, London, p. 245.

Rudramba

With his wide-open eyes, Marco Polo looked at the horses lined up for auction. The various breeds of horses, including Coat Roans, Sorrels, Palominos and others, were impressive. Standing near the platform were the merchants of horses who came from as far as Hormuz, Kais, Dhofar, Shihr and Aden.

'The Arabs buy the best horses and export them here,' Chetti Sadananda told him. Chetti was a horse trader and a mediator for the horse buyers and the Arab merchants. Large-scale horse trade had brought vast fortunes to the merchants and the middlemen.

'Why don't you breed horses here?' Marco had an obvious query.

'There are many reasons which restrict breeding of quality horses here. The climate, soil conditions and natural pasturage are not suitable for the quality horses. Even if we breed, we produce nothing but wretched wry-legged weeds.'

Chetti laughed and then whispered in Marco's ears, 'Isn't good for us? Horses are expensive commodity here. Our kings spend a greater part of their revenue in buying horses. Marco, you should trade in horses. You will reap gold.'

'Don't joke.' Marco replied. He was still curious about this mad craze for the Arabian horses. 'How much do they cost?'

'Look, a good horse is sold in as much as 500 saggi of gold. And, do you know how many the Pandya king buys? Two thousand horses per year. His relatives, ministers and others also buy in huge numbers. But, at the end of the year only a few hundred survive.' Chetti looked gleeful. 'So, next year I import few thousands more...and make more money.'

'How do they die?'

'They buy horses but don't know how to take care of them. We don't have experienced horse breeders.'

'If it is so, why don't the kings import veterinaries?'

'Arabs don't allow it. Traders are happy if the horses die in more numbers.' Chetti smiled cunningly.

Suddenly, a merchant standing nearby said, 'I don't believe this.'

Marco Polo looked at the interrupter and found a stout and well-attired old man. The old man introduced himself as a local trader.

'Sanskrit texts are available on medical treatment of horses and elephants. If the Pandyas can't keep their imported horses well, the blame is on them. Look at the Kakatiyas. Ah, how well they keep their horses. Queen Rudramba of Warangal knows how to maintain a great cavalry.'

Chetti Sadananda kept quiet. But Marco Polo became curious.

'Who is she?' He asked the trader.

'After their dominion in South India for over three centuries, both the Chalukya and the Chola empires disappeared in the beginning of the thirteenth century. On the ruins of these vanished empires, four kingdoms emerged,' the trader began.

'And now they are filling the annals of this century with their mutual hostilities,' Sadananda sarcastically interrupted.

Undeterred by the Chetti's comment, the fellow trader continued.

'These four kingdoms are the Pandya and the Hoysala in south, and the Kakatiya and the Yadava in north. There are few minor powers, such as Telugu-Chodas of Nellore as well. It is true that in the last hundred years there have been no major social or political development, but it is also true that the industry, trade and arts have continued to flourish ...'

'The Queen?' Marco Polo was impatient to know.

The trader did not like this. 'Marco, you first need to know the peninsular politics to appreciate her well.'

Marco Polo apologized and nodded his head in agreement.

Early Kakatiyas were nobles in the courts of the Chalukya kings. Prataparudra I was the first independent Kakatiya king. Once the Chalukya Empire tottered, Prataparudra I founded a new dynasty. In his reign of thirty-eight years, he expanded his kingdom in the entire eastern part of South India, and made Warangal his capital.

At the same time, Bhillam, a former kshatrapa of the Chalukya kings, founded the Yadava dynasty at Devagiri. In 1196, after the death of Bhillam, Jaitugi became the Yadava king. He was constantly in war with his neighbours. In one such war against the Kakatiyas, Jaitugi defeated Prataparudra I and imprisoned his son, Ganapati.

A few months after that war, Prataparudra I died and a

war for ascension to the throne began among the Kakatiya princes. In such a delicate situation, Jaitugi intervened. He released Ganapati from the prison and helped him sit on the Kakatiya throne in 1199. The new ruler Ganapati ruled for more than sixty years and earned the reputation of a good administrator.

Ganapati ruled during the fragile political environment of peninsular India. Unaware of the Turkish danger looming large over their head, the four major kingdoms of South—the Yadavas, the Kakatiyas, the Pandyas and the Hoyasalas—were always at war with each other. The rivalry between Jaitugi's son Singhana and Ganapati became legendary.

During their reign, there was hardly any decade when their kingdoms were not battling each other. However, the result of the wars always remained indecisive.

The disappearance of the power of Velanandi Chodas in the Andhra helped Ganapati to capture and exploit the fertile lands, iron and diamond mines, and ports in coastal Andhra. He also defeated the Telugu-Chodas of Nellore and the king of Kalinga.

Ganapati had two daughters, Rudramba and Ganapamba. Rudramba was the elder daughter. After her birth, the royal astrologer had predicted, 'This girl is blessed by both Mahadeva and Parvati Maa. She will have qualities of both. She will end the demonic reign of the Yadavas.'

A delighted Ganapati named his daughter Rudramba, after Mahadeva and Parvati, and decided to raise her as a warrior princess.

In 1239, Ganapati defeated the Kayasthas in Cuddapah and Kurnool. The Kayasthas were a formidable force under

Gangaya Sahini and his two nephews. Taking this victory as a good omen, Ganapati, who had no male issue, decided to make Rudramba his heir apparent.

The predictions about Rudramba also reached the ears of Singhana, the Yadava king. Singhana's chief astrologer Changadev, a grandson of famous astrologer Bhaskaracharya, was away for some research. Unfortunately, at the same time, Changadev had gone to Pataliputra where he had founded a college for the study of Bhaskaracharya's *Siddhantashiromani* and other works. In his absence, Singhna consulted other astrologers but remained dissatisfied. He sent a messenger to bring back his chief astrologer. Before Changadev could come back to Devagiri, Singhana died.

Young Rudramba was endowed with a great ruler's qualities, but she was a girl. Even though there were other women rulers, it was still a tough battle for Rudramba to make a mark and be accepted as the next in line for the throne.

The people of Warangal were admirers of their young princess's potential. But, her being virtuous was one thing and succeeding her father as a Kakatiya king was another. Ganapati decided to keep influential priests on his side and announced to perform a putrika yagna.

Putrika yagna, literally meaning the yagna for a daughter, was an exceptional yagna performed by a father who generally did not have a male offspring and who wanted to appoint his daughter to perform the customary obsequies after his death. Thus, this yagna used to give the appointed daughters the status of a son.

Amidst the chanting of Vedic mantras and in the presence of the public, Rudramba was formally designated as a son and given the name, Rudradeva Maharaja.

The fellow trader paused.

'Is it so easy? You perform a yagna and the people will accept her as a boy?' Marco Polo asked, puzzled.

'Why not? These ancient ceremonies are approved by ancient scriptures and sanctioned by dharma.'

'That was not the complete truth!' Chetti Sadananda exclaimed. 'In fact, many people opposed and turned against Ganapati for promoting his daughter, even during his life time.'

'But not the people of Warangal,' the fellow trader was not to go down easily.

'Few kshatraps created problems for Ganapati and revolted. They revolted when Rudramba ascended to the throne.' Chetti was on for a debate.

'I shall come to that soon,' the trader said.

After the Yadava king Singhana's death, Ganapati invaded Devagiri. In a fierce battle, Ganapati snatched some territories in the south-western Andhra from Singhana's grandson Krishna. The next few years remained peaceful.

Rudramba helped her father to issue a special charter of security to protect foreign merchants trading at the port of Motupalli, on the coast of Andhra.

'Father, we should take only a fixed duty from the merchants and should guarantee them their security.'

'I agree. It will promote foreign trade,' Ganapati accepted his wise daughter's suggestion.

'We make the finest quality muslin and the best cut diamonds. Instead of employing our soldiers, let the large trade guilds maintain their own force to protect the goods and the factories.'

'A very good idea!' Ganapati was delighted. 'Our soldiers will only supervise and protect the interests of the state.'

Soon, the coastal trade of the elephants, horses, spices, perfumes, precious stones and superior quality textiles expanded exponentially. Rudramba emphasized on a profit-oriented trade and advised to give less importance to the trade of metalwork, jewellery, pottery and salt.

'One day, we have to annex Vengi,' Rudramba said.

'Why do you think so?' Ganapati asked.

'Vengi will give us a substantial seaboard. The profit coming from sea trade will be immense.' Ganapati agreed to do something about it soon.

With the father and the daughter becoming a formidable force, the Kakatiya power was on the rise. Rudramba redesigned Warangal as an enclosed city in a series of circular fortifications.

The city and the power that it encapsulated was largely the planning of Rudramba and the execution of Ganapati.

In the new capital, Rudramba was married to Virabhadra, a Vengi Chalukya prince.

By 1259, Ganapati's health started deteriorating. News of Ganapati's ill health also encouraged neighbouring states to raise their flags against Warangal.

During initial few years of their joint rule, whilst her father was initiating her into the mysteries of the governance, the country was thrown into confusion and disorder.

Jatavarman Sundara Pandya attacked the Kakatiya territories. Ganapati and Rudramba assembled all their feudatories and faced a huge Pandya army at Muttukur, near Nellore. The Pandya army routed a combined Kakatiya army and crushed the morale of Ganapati and Rudramba. To rub salt to their injury, Sundara Pandya performed a virabhisheka, at Nellore, at the end of his campaign.

A few months later, Nellore's prince Manuma Siddhi approached Ganapati for help against his internal enemies. The Kakatiya court poet Tikkana advised the father-daughter duo to help the prince. However, Ganapati vanquished the enemies of Manuma and seated him firmly on the Nellore throne. The might of the Kakatiyas forced the powerful Kadava chieftain Kopperunjinga to acknowledge Ganapati's overlordship.

These wins gave Ganapati some consolation. But, the defeat at Muttukur was a big loss to his prestige. He had also suffered considerable loss of his territory. It slackened his hold over his feudatories and nobles.

'The kshatrapas have become more powerful and are manifesting an increasing tendency to act independently without referring to us first.' Rudramba told her father.

'Rudramba, perhaps I have become too old and feeble to cope with the new situation.' Ganapati said. 'I would like to withdraw from active politics but will be mentoring you from the background, whenever needed.'

Thus, Ganapati gave complete charge of the kingdom to Rudramba and her counsellors.

The early years of Rudramba's reign were marked by troubles created by the rebellious feudatories. Many vassal nayakas were unwilling to pay obeisance to a woman and submit to her authority. They took up arms against her and attempted to throw her off the throne.

Certain other members of the royal household also made a bid for the throne. Prominent among the rebels were the brothers Hariharadeva and Murarideva. The plot was kept a tight secret and therefore the Queen remained clueless till the rebels arrived at the palace gate. Somehow, Annamambikadevi, the wife of Reddy chief Gona Gannaya saved her life and took her out of the royal palace safely. Hariharadeva and Muraraideva captured Warangal and ousted Rudramba from the capital city.

For a few months, Rudramba remained hidden. However, huge public support remained with her. Most of the feudatories, generals and officials remained firmly loyal to her as well. Hariharadeva and Murarideva in frustration started torturing her supporters.

In hiding, Rudramba succeeded in assembling powerful chiefs to her side. The Kayastha chieftains Ambadeva and his brothers Jannigedeva and Tripurari, Recherala Prasaditya and Gannaya met her at a secret place.

'Murari and Harihara are not getting public support. I hear that even the army is divided in their support to them,' Gannaya informed her.

'Ambadeva has assembled three thousand soldiers and five hundred cavalry. Shall we wait for a few more?' Jannigedeva asked.

Prasaraditya and Ambadeva were of the opinion to wait for some more time. But Rudramba was not ready to wait.

'Why should the people suffer more? Let Prasaditya lead the force and attack the fort; I will lead the public to the palace.'

Both the operations were done simultaneously. When Prasaditya launched a furious attack on the fort with his soldiers, Gannaya assembled about three thousand people at the main crossing. The crowd was ecstatic after finding the Queen amidst them. Rudramba addressed them and then riding on a horse, Rudramba led the people's movement to regain her kingdom.

Hariharadeva and Murarideva could not face the army of Rudramba and fled. Prasaditya firmly suppressed the rebellion. In the next one year, Rudramba could successfully track down all the rebels.

But, her problems were hardly over. Before she could have a firm grip over her kingdom, the Yadavas invaded her kingdom again under King Mahadeva. Rudramba and her nayakas put up a defence. A fierce battle took place between the two armies. Rudramba was leading from the front. After a few hours of ferocious fight, it looked as if the Yadavas would be routed. Rudramba's horse was very close to Mahadeva's when the rear flank of the Kakatiya army suddenly buckled under pressure. The Yadava army's sharp arrows had injured Kakatiya elephants, which trampled their own army. Smart Yadava hunters captured many Kakatiya elephants. Rudramba remained fighting alone. Mahadeva and his soldiers surrounded her.

'Rudramba, they call me the uprooter of the stalk of the lotus of the head of Tillingaraya,' said Mahadeva. Rudramba somehow composed herself.

'Mahadeva, I have lost a battle. I am not seeking mercy. You can chop off my head.'

'I have blown away the façade of the great Rudradeva as tempestuous wind blows away the heap of cotton,' the Seuna king noted gleefully.

Rudramba chose not to reply to his boastings.

'Rudramba, battlefields are for warriors. By calling yourself Rudradeva you cannot become a man. I am sparing your life because I do not kill a woman.'

Mahadeva captured her elephants and some of her insignia before sparing her life.

But, before Mahadeva could retreat with his victorious army, Rudramba quickly assembled her force and attacked the enemy. Before a stunned Mahadeva could react and gather himself, Rudramba was back in her fort. An angry Mahadeva laid siege to the Warangal fort.

'We will show the Seunas our might. We will fight till they are defeated,' Rudramba roared.

For fifteen days, the armies of the Yadavas and the Kakatiyas valiantly fought each other. Rudramba destroyed the entire infantry and half the cavalry of Mahadeva.

Fighting inside the walls of the fort, Rudramba almost captured Mahadeva. However, Mahadeva managed to escape. The Kakatiya army pursued the retreating Yadavas up to the walls of the Yadava capital Devagiri.

Unable to withstand the pressure of Rudramba's army near his walls, Mahadeva sued for peace.

'The Yadavas should pay us a crore of gold coins as war indemnity,' she pressed hard.

Seuna Mahadeva had no other choice. He preferred to conclude a treaty with Rudramba.

'This war indemnity will be distributed among our commanders and soldiers,' Rudramba declared amidst her cheering soldiers.

After constructing a pillar in commemoration of her victory, Rudramba returned from Devagiri.

After a decisive victory over the Yadavas, Rudramba marched over the territories of Eastern Chalukyas and the Haihaya chiefs and included Godavari valley and Vengi under her rule.

Vira Rajendra Chola of Nellore was also defeated and became a vassal of Rudramba.

In 1272, Ambadeva, an ambitious and powerful Kayastha chief, succeeded his brother Tripurarideva. These brothers had earlier helped Rudramba to defeat the rebellion of Harihardeva and Murarideva.

'Kayasthas acknowledge our lordship. Why do you say Ambadeva is an errant youth?' Rudramba asked her chief minister.

'He forswears his allegiance to you, Queen. He has resolved to resuscitate the fortunes of his family.'

'So, he wants to carve out an independent kingdom for himself,' Rudramba smiled.

'Should we attack him?'

'No. Until he does not harm our interests, let the man fulfil his dreams first,' Rudramba decided.

However, he came into conflict with the Kakatiya feudatories within few years of his ascension.

One by one, Ambadeva started decimating neighbourhood lords and Kakatiya nayakas. When finally Rudramba decided to act against him, twelve vassal princes and many rulers of neighbouring states were serving Ambadeva. They used to dispatch elephants, horses, costly jewels and other valuable gifts regularly to him.

Ambadeva also entered into an alliance with the Yadavas and the Pandyas, the hereditary foes of the Kakatiyas. Thus, for thirty-two years, Ambadeva constantly remained engaged in warfare with his neighbours. Finally, when he was about to launch an attack on Warangal, Rudramba took few initiatives to stop him.

In Warangal, Rudramba started grooming her grandson Kumara Rudradeva as the next king of the Kakatiyas.

One day she announced, 'Son, now you are ready for the war. Carefully draw your plan for invasion. You should remember that the attack on Ambadeva would also involve you in a war with his allies.'

'I know this, grandmother.'

'Son, your object should be to isolate Ambadeva from his allies and then to deal with each of them separately.'

'How?'

'We will devise a three-pronged attack on Ambadeva's territories and at the same time we will send separate expeditions against his allies,' Rudramba explained her war plans to her grandson.

In 1291, Rudramba, with her huge army, set out for Tripurantakam to attack Ambadeva. In one single onslaught, she captured seventy-two forts and defeated Ambadeva. Ambadeva retreated further south, leaving his capital Tripurantakam and the surrounding country in the hands of Rudramba. A victorious Rudramba quickly put in place many concerted measures to re-establish her authority over the region.

At the same time, her commander Tata Pinnama attacked a powerful local ally of Ambadeva and few battalions of the

Kakatiya army attacked Nellore. Simultaneously, another expedition was set out against the Yadavas.

Rudramba, thus, conquered the entire Krishna-Tungbhadra doab and defeated her enemies comprehensively.

As a result of these victories, the Kaktiyas emerged as the greatest power in the peninsula.

After securing her kingdom's boundaries, Rudramba focused on the administration and foreign trade.

Her conduct of affairs fully justified the trust her father reposed at her. Attired in male garments, she daily presided over the durbar, invited foreigners to her land to write about it, held consultations with her ministers, generals and other high officers of the state and advised all these how they should act to promote the best interests of the state.

On occasions of emergency, she did not hesitate to lead her troops against the enemy. And, in spite of the wars which frequently disturbed her country, her people remained contended and happy under her rule.

The fellow trader paused and then informed Marco Polo.

'Marco, I don't know any other country where so many methods are used to gather diamonds from the mines. We make the best and the most delicate buckrams and the costliest. If you see them, they look like tissues of a spider's web. Marco, you must buy them. There is no king or queen in the world who will not be glad to wear them. In Rudramba's reign, you won't find any scarcity; we all have great abundance of all the necessities of life.'

'I would like to visit one of those places.' Marco said

genuinely. 'Is the conflict with the Yadavas over forever?'

'No. The hostility continues. In fact, the Queen is very old now. Ramchandra attacked Warangal again and recently the Queen sent her other grandson Prataparudradeva to crush the Yadavas. Prataparudradeva won the decisive battle and crushed the Yadavas.'

The trader paused before adding, 'Life plays strange games, foreigner. In politics, no foe or friend is permanent. Look how, the Kayastha chieftain, Ambadeva, who so gallantly helped Rudramba to regain her throne, rebelled later.'

That was in 1292. Much later, when he started writing about his visit to South India, Marco Polo had gathered more knowledge about the Kakatiyas and Rudramba, whom she called 'a lady of much discretion'. She ruled till 1295 and then passed the baton to Prataparudradeva. Till her death, she kept on guiding the young king. As a result, Kuntala and the forts of Adoni and Raichur came under Prataparudra's control. The Yadava garrisons in Andhra were destroyed or brought under control of the Kakatiyas. The young king worked on the administrative model developed by Rudramba and reformed the system by dividing his kingdom into seventy-seven nayakships. This great reformative system was later adopted and elaborated by the rulers of Vijayanagar.

Rudramba encouraged a strong cavalry and ensured that the horses were well taken care of. As a result, when Ala-ud-din Khalji's huge army attacked them, the Kakatiya cavalry defeated the Sultanate army.

'The Kakatiya army defeated Khalji?' The statement surprised Marco Polo's disciple.

'Yes.' Marco replied gleefully. 'In 1303, Ala-ud-din sent a

huge army under the command of Fakhr-ud-din Jauna, Delhi's present sultan, Muhammad Bin Tughlaq.'*

Marco's pride was evident. 'That year, Muhammad Tughlaq came to invade Warangal taking a route through Orissa. But, the campaign failed disastrously. His army had to suffer a humiliating defeat in Warangal, and had to retreat in disarray.'

---

*Ghazi Malik, or Ghiyasuddin Tughlaq, was the father of Muhammad Bin Tughluq and was a provincial governor under the Khiljis. Fakhr-ud-din Jauna, as Muhammad was known before his coronation, had led expeditions under Ala-ud-din's reign.

Durgavati

On top of a carefully erected machan, masterful, calm and equable, Mihirunnisa was sitting very close to Jahangir, the Mughal emperor. Bows, arrows and newly acquired guns were kept neatly arranged in front of them. The sun had already set and darkness was engulfing with every passing second. She could see the departing sun's weak rays bidding goodbye to the equally weak waves of the pond. The pond, where wild animals would visit later in the night, was about forty to fifty feet open from all sides.

Jahangir looked towards the west, and then at Mihirunnisa. 'Masha Allah! She is beautiful!,' he thought and kept looking at her face. Sher Afgan's vivacious, vital and energetic wife had already stolen his heart—why else would the Emperor be sitting with her in this dense forest, waiting for the tigers?

With her large and lustrous eyes, broad forehead, sharp nose, strong chin, and small but well formed lips, and a hint of a smile playing at their corners, Mihirunnisa had captivated Jahangir.

That day, Jahangir was keen on testing her shooting skills.

When in the morning she heard Jahangir was going hunting, Mihirunnisa had requested him to take her along.

Initially, he was not enthusiastic on taking his lover on the hunt. Father of the richly talented Mihirunnisa, the witty Itimad-ud-daula, tried to convince him.

'Shahenshah, she can take care of herself in the jungle. She is an excellent shot.'

Jahangir laughed, 'I know only one lady who could kill a tiger in one shot—the Queen Durgavati of Gondwana.'

When a speechless Mihirunnisa raised her eyebrows sharply, Jahangir decided not to displease his lady love.

Detailed arrangements were made for the royal safari. Mihirunnisa refused to sit on an elephant and instead rode a white horse by her paramour's side.

'Who is Durgavati?'

'She was the queen of Gondwana and died fighting Asaf Khan in 1564.'

'Was she a great shot?'

'Better than many of us. She could kill a tiger with one arrow. The moment she knew any tiger was in the vicinity, she would abandon everything and rush to hunt the beast. A great hunting enthusiast, a brave queen, and what a ruler!'

Her beloved's generous words for someone else filled Mihirunnisa's heart with jealousy. She urged Jahangir to tell her more about Durgavati.

'Nur, have you heard about the great Hindu temples of Khajuraho?'

'What is the relationship between a Gond Durgavati and the elite Chandels?'

'She was the bridge between the Gonds and the Chandels. She was a Chandel princess and a Gond queen.'

'The Fort of Kalinjar in Bundelkhand was considered an

impregnable fort. Even my grandfather Humayun could not win the fort. It was invincible and the King Kirat Singh was resolute. Sher Shah Suri conquered it after a year long siege, but he had to pay for his life. Durgavati was the daughter of Kirat Singh Chandel. The Chandels were very proud of their lineage and tradition, and Kirat Singh was no different.

'Kirat Singh had proposed Durgavati's marriage to several Kshatriya princes of reputed lineage. However, Durgavati turned down every proposal.'

'Why?' A surprised Mihirunnisa asked.

'The supremely talented Durgavati wanted to marry a person who could match her qualities.' Thus, Jahangir began Queen Durgavati's fascinating life story.

When Princess Durgavati's favourite maid Ramcheri told her about Prince Dalpat Shah of Gondwana, her curiosity and affection were aroused.

'Princess, I saw him in Maniyagarh where he had killed a notorious man-eater. He is your match in tiger hunting. His smile is intoxicating and his innocent face is so attractive. Riding on a black horse with a huge bow on his shoulder, the tall and handsome Gond prince looked like Lord Ram,' Ramcheri explained.

When Kirat Singh began heavily insisting on marriage, Durgavati decided to tell her father about her choice, albeit indirectly.

'Dalpat Shah?' her father smiled. 'One in a million! He is a brave, wise and a very handsome prince,' said Kirat Singh before suddenly appearing pensive.

'Durga, Gondwana, or Garha Katanga, is a huge state. Prosperous people, large tracts of land full of crops, huge hills, many forts and abundance of minerals! Thousands of lakes—big and small! Wild animals and wilderness on one side and thousands of brave soldiers on the other! What a powerful country it is. But, they are Gonds and we are Chandels. Dalpat may be a prosperous royal but he is a tribal king and we, Durga, are true royal blood kshatriyas.'

The princess kept quiet for some time.

'Father, today Humayun and Sher Shah are fighting for the throne of Hindustan. Whosoever wins, will attack us next. We are surrounded by small, selfish and visionless kingdoms and only an alliance with the powerful Gonds can save us from the Mughals or Pathans.'

'Durga, how can I give you away to a Gond just for my selfish gains?'

'Father, don't view Prince Dalpat through a narrow lens of caste. This caste system has decimated our society. We are not ready to share our food with the Gonds and we leave no chance to humiliate our own brethren. That is precisely the reason why a handful of outsiders have succeeded in demolishing us all.'

Kirat Singh knew this very well. The power and prestige of the Raj-Gonds was no less than the Chandels. The fear of social backlash was the only reason Kirat Singh was not agreeing to Durgavati's wish. He said, 'If tomorrow the Afghans or the Mughals attack us, only our combined force can vanquish them. But...'

'But what will our people say? All of them—the Chandels, Baghels, Chauhans and Rajputs—will oppose us.'

Durgavati did not reply, but she refused to give up.

She proposed to invite Dalpat Shah for a hunting expedition. Goddess Maniya Devi was considered to be an incarnation of the goddess Durga, and both the Chandels and the Gonds worshipped her. Annually, the local people organized a huge festival on a full moon night in the month of Agrahan at Maniyagarh. Durgavati somehow convinced Kirat Singh to invite Dalpat Shah for a hunting expedition during this festival. Dalpat agreed to the proposal, as he was curious to meet Durgavati himself.

The two days at Maniyagarh provided an opportunity to the couple to know each other well. Together they hunted tigers and participated in other festivities. Durgavati found Dalpat to be a charming, courageous and wise person. Love blossomed on both sides and Kirat Singh knowingly looked away.

Though Kirat Singh was afraid of the infamy derived from an alliance with Dalpat, he was under no illusion—the once glorious Chandel kingdom was now limited to Mahoba and Kalinjar, with only 3,000 soldiers, 2,000 cavaliers and 25 elephants. His only hope was the invincible fort of Kalinjar.

In 1543, when Kirat Singh went to inspect Mahoba for few days, Durgavati slipped out of the fort one night through a secret tunnel. After coming out of the tunnel, she walked for a few miles to reach the place of their rendezvous. A smiling Dalpat and a few of his riders were waiting for her.

They got married at the fort of Singaurgarh, the capital of Gondwana. The Gonds welcomed their queen with great pomp and show.

After the wedding, Duragavati and Dalpat Shah took a tour of their kingdom. Dalpat bestowed equal status upon Durgavati but many including Chandra Singh, his younger brother, did not like it.

When Durgavati called upon volunteers for a public cleaning exercise, Chandra Singh objected.

'Bhabhiji, you should not go in public.'

'Why?'

'Because in our home, women follow the purdah system.'

'Purdah in Gondwana?'

'The Gonds don't follow it but we Rajgonds do.'

Durgavati laughed. 'Sanskritisation is useful if we imbibe the positive elements of a powerful culture. Why should we acquire their bad practices? I will not follow the purdah.'

Ignoring the anger on Chandra Singh's face, Durgavati asked, 'Who has asked you to convey this to me?'

'No one.'

'I won't take order from anyone, unless it is decreed by the king.'

The message spread quickly. The public welcomed it, though the palace remained cautious. Knowing very well how much the king loved her, no one could openly oppose her decision.

'Maharaj, how did you get this Mussulman title of "Shah"?' Durgavati asked Dalpat Shah one day.

'I inherited the title. Once Jalaluddin Lodi, younger brother of Dilli's Sultan Ibrahim Lodi, revolted. When chased by the Sultanate forces, he came to our fort Chauragarh with his army and requested shelter and protection. My father, King Sangram Singh wisely decided not to annoy the Sultan of Dilli and fought against Jalaluddin's army and arrested him. Later, he deported him to Dilli. A pleased Sultan conferred the title of Shah on my father and started calling him Sangram Shah.'

In 1545, when Durgavati was pregnant, Garha Katanga got threats from the neighbouring sultans of Sarangpur and Malwa. Sher Shah marched towards Kalinjar with a huge army. Before Kirat Singh could send a message to Dalpat Shah, Sher Shah had attacked Kalinjar. But contrary to the Afghan army's expectations, the siege dragged on for nearly a year.

Despite the betrayal of one of his closest commanders, Kirat Singh defended his fort admiringly. Finally, when the trenches could not be used anymore, Sher Shah built an observation tower close to the fort, which facilitated the Afghans to gun down the people in the fort with muskets. One morning, when Sher Shah came down to supervise the rocket launching into the fort, one of the rockets hit the fort wall and recoiled with great force and exploded, burning him severely from head to toe.

Severely injured, Sher Shah remained fitfully conscious. Between consciousness he shouted to his men encouraging them to seize the fort. In the afternoon, he died after hearing of the fall of the fort and the arrest of Kirat Singh. Dying with the satisfaction of having won the fort, he ordered the death for Kirat Singh.

When the news of the fall of Kalinjar and demise of Kirat Singh reached Singaurgarh, Durgavati had just given birth to her son, Vir Narayan. For many days, she mourned her father's death. He was her mentor and unrivaled supporter.

'I shall forever follow the path shown by him and shall never shun my duties and responsibilities,' she vowed.

Inspired by Durgavati, Dalpat Shah took new initiatives in irrigation, agriculture and construction of roads; later he rationalized his tax collection policies. The citizens were happy and the royal couple was busy in serving them.

But cruel fate had other designs. In 1548, Dalpat Shah fell ill and despite the best available treatment, never recovered and passed away. Patiently, Durgavati arranged for the funeral of her beloved husband, but her brother-in-law had other designs.

'We follow the practice of sati. Rani Ma must prepare for that,' Chandra Singh announced.

'I am not sure. Vir Narayan is only three years old,' Ramcheri replied.

'So what? I can take care of him as well as the kingdom,' Chandra Singh said.

'You better ask the Queen.' Ramcheri loathed the ambitious Chandra Singh.

'Rani Ma, what will happen now?' Chandra Singh asked the Queen.

'We will run the administration. We will take care of Vir,' said Durgavati fully aware of what Chandra Singh had in mind.

'I heard that you don't want to follow brother Dalpat to heaven. We, Rajgonds, follow the tradition of sati,' Chandra Singh sounded solemn.

'Chandra Singh, for me, the interests of the kingdom and my son Vir come before following the tradition.'

When the customary mourning period got over, Vir Narayan was coronated as the king of Garha Katanga under the patronage of Durgavati.

Chandra Singh objected to it.

'How is it possible for a widow to sit in the open and run the kingdom?'

During a heated discussion, Durgavati cleared the air, 'Purdah and silence are not for me. I am accustomed to sit in an open durbar. I have a right to opinion in matters related to the kingdom, my son and myself.'

'This will bring infamy to our dynasty,' Chandra Singh protested.

'Evil acts bring infamy to a clan. You do whatever you feel is right,' Durgavati said sternly.

'In that case, I have no option but to leave the kingdom,' Chandra Singh threatened.

'If that makes you happy, I will not stop you. This kingdom belongs to your brother and nephew, you are always welcome here.'

Chandra Singh did not wait further and stomped out of the court.

Without wasting any time, Durgavati completely absorbed herself in the matters of running the kingdom. With the intent of welfare and the prosperity of her people in mind, she audited the royal treasury, inspected official documents, made policies and appointed suitable officers to implement them.

To know her people and the kingdom better, Durgavati started statewide tours. First she visited the places close to the enemy kingdoms and made necessary arrangements to build a stronger defence system. New ponds were dug and old ponds were revitalized, embankments were reinforced, handicraft was promoted, and bell metal and iron works were encouraged. Maintenance of the forts at Chauragarh, Garha, Varahvan, Patan and Hariyagarh were started.

'Rani Ma, these plans will empty the royal treasure,' Minister Adhar Singh said.

'What else is the use of such treasure?'

'For any emergency, Rani Ma.'

'In that case, let us keep a small portion for an emergency and spend the rest on people's welfare. If people are in distress, we should first spend on them.'

'Very well,' said Adhar Singh and then quickly changed the topic to appease the Queen.

'Rani Ma, the Garha jungles have many tigers.'

'No, Adhar Singh, I have given up hunting. I should concentrate on governance.'

The Queen kept on visiting places, meeting people and directing welfare works.

Meanwhile, news arrived that Baj Bahadur of Malwa was planning to attack Garha. With an army double the size of Gondwana's army, he, along with his uncle, Fateh Khan, approached Garha. But the wise Queen took her army many miles northwest of Garha, where the only route to reach Garha was through a pass between two big hills. She deployed her archers on the two hilltops and kept her elephants in the rear.

The Queen patiently allowed the entire army of Baj Bahadur to enter inside the long pass. A rain of arrows from the hilltops pierced the limbs of Malwa's soldiers. In the ensuing mayhem, Fateh Khan was killed but Baj Bahadur somehow slipped away.

Despite this humiliating defeat, an undeterred Baj Bahadur kept attacking Gondwana but was defeated each time by the Queen.

Assuming Durgavati's army had grown tired and weaker after the successive wars with Malwa, the Sultan of Beeder attacked Gondwana.

But the Queen was ready for the eminent attack. She positioned her army on a huge plain ahead of the hills. She kept her elephants at the front and the cavalry behind them. Her cavalry was well protected with iron shields. When the Sultan attacked, after a little show of resistance, the Gondwana elephants dispersed and the horses withdrew into the hills.

Looking at his retreating enemy, an elated Sultan threw away all his caution to the wind. Chasing the recoiling Gondwana soldiers, his army entered the valley and fell into the trap. An incessant shower of poisonous arrows drenched the Beeder army and its horrified soldiers looked for an escape, but the Queen's elephants had blocked all exit points. The Beeder army was captured and only the Sultan could manage a disgraceful escape.

'That's incredible. So could she live peacefully thereafter?' Mihirunnisa asked.

'No,' Jahangir was in pensive mood. 'Baj Bahadur kept on attacking Gondwana for the next six years but never succeeded. In the year 1562, Abba Huzur's army attacked Malwa and vanquished Baj Bahadur, thereby bringing Malwa under the Mughal dominion.'

'So, Gondwana's boundary touched that of the mighty Mughals.'

'Absolutely, Nur,' Jahangir said. 'Malwa's defeat made a significant change in the fate of Gondwana.'

'Emperor Akbar's cherished dream was to bring all of Hindustan under one umbrella. Abba Huzur had heard a lot about the prosperity of the Gondwana kingdom and the personality of Durgavati. He deputed Asaf Khan to deal with the Queen,' Jahangir said.

Khwaja Abdul Majid Asaf Khan was a highly ambitious Mughal general. After vanquishing Ramchandra, the ruler of Rewa, he was determined to win all neighbouring states. Thus, he went to Emperor Akbar and sought permission to deal with Gondwana. Akbar happily obliged him.

Asaf Khan sent his messenger with a letter and a golden cage to the court of Durgavati.

'Your majesty, a beautiful woman like you is not meant to suffer the rugged chores of the governance. For her own safety, a beautiful bird should live in a golden cage. We will take care of you. Else, when our canons boom, you won't find a single Gond alive.'

This message made the Queen furious. Since the message was written in the name of Akbar, Durgavati replied to the emperor and not to Asaf Khan. She sent him a golden *pinjan*, an instrument used to ginning or bowing cotton.

'Raja Akbar,' her message read, 'you are not fit to rule. It's better you bow cotton.'

This terse reply made the emperor furious and he permitted Asaf Khan to go ahead and attack Gondwana. From Malwa, Asaf Khan reached Maniyagarh and began an unending spell of arson, massacre and loot until he reached the northern hills of Damoh. He stationed his army on these hills and sent a few huntsmen out in the open; the famed Mughal canons were kept safely in the hills. Asaf Khan was alert and taking every necessary precaution.

On the other hand, Durgavati moved vigilantly but quickly. She reached a place near the Bhander and Kaimur hills. Her fast pace only allowed her to bring along 500 soldiers, but she set them intelligently. The elephants were left behind near the passes and a portion of the archers was stationed there. With a hundred cavaliers, she moved from one side of the hill along a rivulet. Asaf Khan was just across the hills and saw the Queen approaching, and the battle began. The archers from both the sides were unrivaled but the Mughals had the advantage of guns. After a short skirmish, Durgavati withdrew her force and retreated on the same path along the rivulet.

When the Mughals saw the Queen withdrawing, they chased her. Durgavati and her horsemen were retreating while defending themselves. When they reached the hills, where the stream was narrower and the hills closer, they found themselves under the Gond arrows. Before the Mughals could understand what was happening, they were trapped. Many of them were killed but many more kept coming in—valiantly shooting arrows and firing their guns. The Queen's soldiers held their position gallantly. As a result, the rate of casualties in the Mughal army kept growing steadily. Sensing that, Asaf Khan signalled his men to retreat.

The victorious force of the Queen had also suffered huge casualties. She returned to Singaurgarh with her injured soldiers.

The northern hills of Damoh were still under the control of Asaf Khan. The Queen sent a few hundred men to reinforce the contingent deployed in the Bhander and Kaimur hills. She also reinforced the defence of Singaurgarh and stocked huge quantities of grains inside the fort. In the next following days, many little skirmishes took place between the two armies. Each time, the Mughals lost and suffered huge casualties. Despite that, thanks to his large army, Asaf Khan approached Singaurgarh slowly and surely. The Mughal army was huge and a few hundred casualties could not deter them.

Finally, Asaf Khan succeeded in capturing the neighbouring hills of Singaurgarh. Despite the stiff resistance, the Mughals managed to station their guns on top of the hills. This deterred the Queen's guerilla tactics. Singaurgarh remained under siege for more than a month. Ration was now growing scarce and the enemy had blocked every entrance to the fort. Before the attack of the Mughals, Durgavati had allocated parts of her army to defend the forts of Chauragarh, Garha and Patan. She planned to leave Singaurgarh if it fell into enemy hands.

Asaf Khan was a smart general. Outsmarting the Queen, he cordoned off all the routes out of Singaurgarh by deploying agile horsemen—especially on roads leading to Chauragarh, Garha and Patan.

A trapped Durgavati considered her options and took a daring step: at night, she quietly came out of the fort with about fifty swordsmen and ten cavaliers and moved closer to the Mughal camp stationed to secure the route to Patan. She left her horses at a fair distance. The surprise attack stunned the Mughal soldiers. The sword fight lasted only thirty minutes and the entire Mughal contingent was slayed. The Queen signalled her horsemen to follow the plan. In no time, the entire population of Singaurgarh was brought out on the road and sent to Garha and Patan. Though the Mughals had a large army, the topography of the hills was unknown to them. This allowed the Queen to safely arrive at Garha, with minimal loss.

This incident made a huge dent in Asaf Khan's prestige. After capturing Singaurgarh, he attacked Garha without taking a break. Durgavati decided to move to Chauragarh. But the incessant rains made the River Narmada swell up due to which the Queen had to halt on its banks with 3,000 soldiers.

Asaf Khan sniffed out her location and sent his troops to fortify all the escape routes to Bheraghat, Barela and Mahishmati. Vir Narayan and Durgavati attacked the Mughal camps at Bheraghat and Mahishmati simultaneously and overpowered them after a daylong skirmish. In the evening, both the chunks of Durgavati's army met on the bank of Narmada. Everyone was tired but the Queen cautioned them.

'Tomorrow, the Mughal canons will get here and the battle may draw longer. Let's attack the Mughals at Barela.'

No one moved including Vir Narayan. Everyone was tired and longed for a night's rest.

'Ma, the army is tired and the soldiers are wounded. Let us rest for now. At dawn, we will attack,' Vir Narayan requested.

Durgavati stayed awake through the night and woke her army up before the crack of dawn. But as daylight broke, to their horror, they saw the Mughals ready for an attack. A fierce battle commenced, where Vir Narayan was injured. The Queen arranged for his safe escape and plunged into the fight herself. The Mughal soldiers were getting closer and the large Mughal army was about to swallow the Queen and her archers. Suddenly, an arrow pierced the Queen's right temple. She pulled it out with force but its head remained pinned inside. She kept on fighting but with sagging breath. Soon, another arrow pierced through her neck and she fell off her elephant.

'Pass me your dagger. I shall not allow the enemy to capture me alive,' she commanded her mahout. He hesitated for a while and then passed the dagger.

Enthralled and mesmerized, Mihirunnisa could do nothing that night except listen to the story and later watch Jahangir kill a leopard. The story of Durgavati kept on reverberating in her ears. She vowed to replicate the feat of the brave Queen of Gondwana.

Since then, Mihirunnisa, who later came to be known as Nur-e-Jahan, never missed any opportunity to accompany Jahangir in his hunting expeditions. As a result, she became an excellent shot and once felled four tigers in six shots.

Until now, such shooting was never seen—from the top of an elephant and inside of a howdah, six arrows were shot killing four beasts that found no opportunity to spring or move. An exalted Jahangir rewarded Nur-e-Jahan with a pair of diamond bracelets, and also showered 1,000 gold ashrafis over her.

Chand Bibi

'Have you read the Queen's Proclamation?' Philip Meadows Taylor asked his wife, Mary Palmer. It was a quiet Sunday morning in November, 1858.

Taylor looked at his beautiful Eurasian wife—she was the granddaughter of William Palmer, the East India Company's Resident at Hyderabad. Her grandmother was one of the princesses of the Royal House of Delhi.

'Yes, Victoria is now the queen of India, as well as of the United Kingdom. The great rebellion has been crushed and the fictitious Company rule is finally over. We will no longer be usurping native states following an unscrupulous doctrine, and yes, the queen's rule will put an end to any plan to rapidly transform the so called savage natives.'

The moment he uttered the words, Taylor knew that his wife would be very upset.

'The great rebellion will not prove to be a disaster, Philip,' Mary said coldly. 'It will inspire a new kind of rebellion that will end this unjust British dominion over India.'

'I don't agree,' Taylor politely disagreed. 'Mary, a small company of Queen Elizabeth defeated the mighty Mughals in the past. Now under Queen Victoria's rule, on which the sun never sets, such a rebellion by the natives is impossible. Leave aside the talk of Her Highness, India never even had a match for the witty Queen Elizabeth.'

'Philip, ignorance breeds arrogance. You know very little about the Indian history,' Mary challenged her husband.

'Tell me, could any Indian king match Queen Elizabeth?' Taylor was not the one to go down without a fight. He had been a highly successful administrator, an expert on megaliths, law, geology and Indian antiquities. He had also worked as a judge, an engineer, an artiste, and was a man of letters. His novel *Confessions of a Thug* had become very popular.

'Philip, I will not talk about the great Mughals but will tell you about a lady regent. Few in England know about this princess of Deccan, who was contemporary to Queen Elizabeth and was equal to her in political talent, though in a different sense. She was well educated and accomplished, and ruled over a population as large and rich as England; a woman who was surrounded by jealous enemies but preserved her kingdom from destruction and partition with valour and endurance. She exercised absolute power but was also simple, generous, frank, chaste, virtuous, religious and charitable. She was a jewel without a flaw and beyond comparison.'

'Who was she?' Philip had never heard about such a princess.

'Chand Bibi, the princess of Ahmednagar, a Deccan kingdom.'

'I have heard her name but what was so extraordinary about her that you compare her to Queen Elizabeth?' Philip probed further.

In the fourteenth century, in Deccan, two very powerful kingdoms emerged from the the remains of the Khalji conquests in the peninsula—the Vijayanagar and Bahmanid kingdoms. The kings of Vijayanagar were Hindus and are often credited for spearheading Hindu resistance against the Islamic rule in the peninsula. On the other hand, Hasan and his Brahmin master Gangu founded the Muslim Bahmanid kingdom. For the next two centuries, the two empires fought with each other to gain supremacy in the south. The main issue of conflict between them was a rich tract of land, between the Krishna and Tungabhadra rivers, known as the Raichur Doab.

This peril compelled them to remain at war, forever. Around the end of the fifteenth century, the Bahmanid kingdom disintegrated into four powerful Muslim states—Ahmednagar, Bijapur, Berar, and Golkunda. But, their internal fights and their war with Vijayanagar continued. There were times when these states even took help from Vijayanagar in the wars against each other.

Chand Bibi was the daughter of Husain Nizam Shah, the Sultan of Ahmednagar. She was the apple of the eye of the royal Nizam Shahi family.

In those days, Ali Adil Shah, the Sultan of Bijapur was very close to Ram Raya, the king of Vijayanagar. However, when Ram Raya's men plundered Ahmednagar twice, the alliance collapsed. The dominance and the prestige of Ram Raya in Deccan forced all four of his enemies to come together against him.

Between the years 1564 and 1565, these four Deccan

states entered into close matrimonial and political alliances, with the intention of ending the supremacy of Vijayanagar. To cement the bond of friendship, Husain Nizam Shah, the Sultan of Ahmednagar agreed to give his daughter, Chand Bibi in marriage to Ali Adil Shah, the Sultan of Bijapur with the fort of Sholapur as dowry. In return, it was arranged that Adil Shah would give the hand of his sister to Murtaza, a son of Husain Nizam Shah, whose second daughter was married to the king of Golkunda.

These double marriages were celebrated in Bijapur and Ahmednagar with joy. For Adil Shah, Chand Bibi was a prize more valuable than many forts. She was extremely beautiful, suave, well-versed in the art of administration, an excellent archer and a deft rider.

'What happened to Vijayanagar?' Philip asked.

'The grand alliance rang the bells of doom for Vijayanagar. Despite old Rama Raya's valour, his huge army was defeated by the Deccan alliance in 1565 at Rakshas-Tangadi, and the city of Vijayanagar was plundered and ruined by the confederacy.'

'So, Chand Bibi ruled Bijapur after her husband?'

'No. Ahmednagar,' Mary corrected him.

Taylor looked at his wife in confusion. Mary smiled and said, 'Philip, the grand victory over Vijayanagar affected the most ambitious winners differently.'

After his arduous campaign, the Sultan of Ahmednagar needed rest and relaxation. Husain Nizam Shah took to drinking and enjoying the company of beautiful damsels and cheerful wine cupbearers. As a result, his health gave away so fast that he died within six months of his famed victory.

After his father's death, Murtaza Nizam Shah became the sultan of Ahmednagar. During his reign, the nobles in the court became very powerful and wars among the members of the confederacy became a norm.

In 1580, Ali Adil Shah was assassinated in Bijapur. This murder brought about a change in the entire political situation in Deccan. Ibrahim Adil Shah, his successor, was merely a child of nine. Chand Bibi guided him with wisdom and valour, but she was surrounded by jealous and highly ambitious nobles.

In Ahmednagar, with the passage of time, Murtaza became a self-indulgent and licentious debauch. As a result, the nobles became more influential than the sultan. Murtaza died in 1588, and with that ended the glorious rise of the Ahmednagar kingdom. Before his death, lowborn ruffians, who had crept into the politics of the kingdom, began to play the role of kingmakers. Thus, after the death of Murtaza, began an era of chaos and confusion, of massacres and bloodshed which ate into the vital resources of the state, and opened the way for the Mughals to enter Deccan.

After the death of Murtaza, hostilities among the Deccanies, Abyssinians, Mahdavis and the foreigners resulted in destruction of property of thousands of people. Whichever group came to power, ordered general massacre of every rank of the other groups, and plundered and burnt their dwellings. On few occasions, the rival nobles were paraded through the streets of the city on donkeys or their mutilated bodies were displayed in public. Sultans were used as pawns, changed at will and even murdered by the powerful nobles. As a result, Ahmednagar spiralled faster towards the path of civil war and self-destruction.

Chand Bibi was worried. Her father's state, Ahmednagar, as well as her husband's Sultanate, Bijapur, were in chaos.

She lamented to her loyal noble, Mustafa.

'Mustafa, in these evil days of general massacre and plundering in Ahmednagar, I feel as if peace and security have vanished. Those who held their heads as high as the heavens with pride are now humbled to dust. Our chaste virgins, who have never shown their faces to sun or to the moon, are dragged by their hair into the bazaar for the pleasures of the drunken men. Buildings which once stood erect to heaven now bow their heads in shame.'

'How did Chand Bibi fare after her husband's death?' Philip intervened.

'Chand Bibi assumed the direction of the state affairs. Even when her husband was alive, she accompanied him on the conquests, riding by his side in the battle field.'

'And in times of peace?'

'She used to address the public and handle business transactions in the open durbar. She oversaw many public projects and the people loved her—not only for her courage and boldness, but also for her sense of justice and firmness.'

'Then?'

'Things went wrong when Kamil Khan became the peshwa and wakil of Bijapur. He began to behave insolently towards her. His outrageous and brutal conduct went on increasing and soon crossed all boundaries of decency.'

'How preposterous!' Philip remarked. 'She should have thrown him out.'

'Remember, Philip. She was a Muslim aristocrat widow in her late husband's Sultanate, which was continuously at loggerheads with her brother's kingdom. It was not easy for her. Once Kamil Khan sent a female slave of the royal harem to her.'

'Kanija, go to Chand Bibi's chamber and molest her. She must be missing her husband's company,' a wicked Kamil Khan directed his slave.

The slave slipped in to the private chambers of Chand Bibi at night and tried to molest her. When Chand Bibi protested the assault and assembled her supporters in palace, Kamil Khan got her arrested for false charge of debauchery. He also started defaming her.

After a few days, he ordered her to leave the palace and proceed to her parental home.

'Kamil, this is too much. Don't you dare say this to me again. This is my kingdom.'

'Bibi, you are the daughter of our enemies. You have to go.'

'Fear my brother, Murtaza. If he hears about this, he will kill you in a moment,' an enraged Chand Bibi threatened her Peshwa.

'How dare you threaten me in the name of your brother? I'll get you beaten up,' Kamil Khan thundered, shaking with anger.

In Bijapur, things had turned worse. It was suffering from

the miserable disease of factional feuds. The dominance of Kamil Khan had become unbearable and Chand Bibi called her noble servant to seek help from another noble, Kishwar Khan.

'Mustafa, go to Haji Kishwar Khan and ask for help.' She sent some cotton and a spinning wheel for the Haji.

'Tell the Haji that the devil has come upon us. If he possesses a grain of self-respect, he should consider my humiliation to be his own. Ask him to blow the brains out of the arrogant Kamil Khan, for making me go through this sea of trouble.' Chand Bibi paused and added, 'Mustafa, remind him the rank and dignity which was once enjoyed by his father and him. Tell him that Chand Bibi will ensure he gets his rightful place in the court again. If he keeps the struggle, the royal family and its well-wishers will be on his side. If not, he should put his hand to the cotton and charkha.'

Sensing his chances, Kishwar Khan acted fast and overthrew Kamil Khan. Chand Bibi kept her word and appointed him as peshwa and wakil.

Unfortunately, Kishwar Khan proved to be no different. After gathering power, he also began to behave like Kamil Khan and started coercing the Queen. Thus, their relationship soured owing to his arrogance and high-handedness.

One morning, Chand Bibi came to know that Kishwar Khan had murdered his loyal noble Sayyid Mustafa Khan. In a fit of rage, she immediately summoned the Peshwa and sought an explanation.

'How dare you murder Mustafa without any allegations? Who are you? Are you a king?'

Kishwar Khan's silence added fuel to fire. Chand Bibi publicly admonished her Peshwa.

'Kishwar Khan, your rank and honour is on the mercy of Adil Shahi Sultanate. Today you are the Peshwa, tomorrow you may be a prisoner.'

Kishwar Khan first recoiled like a serpent and then, watching his men surround the Queen, raised his hood.

'Arrest her,' he ordered his men. 'She has invited her brother to invade Bijapur.'

A stunned Queen looked around, but no one came forward in her support.

'Take her to the fort of Satara and imprison her there.' Kishwar Khan had come with a definite plan.

The shocked people of Bijapur resented the arrest and imprisonment of Chand Bibi and expressed their displeasure by openly abusing Kishwar Khan while he was riding through the city.

Meanwhile, the imprisoned Chand Bibi sent a message to the African amirs seeking their help. They immediately came with their armies to her aid.

An alerted Kishwar Khan, meanwhile, abducted the young king and took him out of Bijapur on the pretext of a hunting excursion. But, soon he realized the futility of opposing the Africans and fled with 400 supporters to Ahmednagar. Chand Bibi ensured that he was not given shelter there, and he was forced to flee to Golkunda. Later, he was caught and slayed there for the murder of Sayyid Mustafa Khan.

When Chand Bibi returned to Bijapur with due honours, even she found it difficult to control the fighting amirs. She was also being accused of being partial to the foreigners. A period of great dissension in Bijapur started, which encouraged the neighbouring kingdoms to relaunch their campaigns against

Bijapur, fired on by their ambitious designs.

In 1595, Chand Bibi's brother and the Sultan of Ahmednagar, Burhan Nizam Shah, fell ill and suffered from chronic dysentery, which confined him to bed. Chand Bibi rushed to her ailing brother's side.

'Chand, I wish I could go and suppress Ismail's rebellion,' Burhan expressed his helplessness to her.

'I shudder to think of Mahdavis' terror returning to Ahmednagar,' Chand Bibi commented. Burhan Shah was a staunch Shia. In a fractured society like Ahmednagar where people were divided among Deccanies, Abyssinians, Mahdavies, Marathas, Sunnies and Shiyas, communal violence was a common thing. Early in his reign, Burhan had abolished the Mahdavi religion and put to death all those who practised it, and reintroduced the Shia faith in Ahmednagar.

Ismail was a rebel and a strict Mahdavi, and was a sworn enemy of the Shias. Supported by the Deccani leaders, he was a potential threat to Ahmednagar's Shia Nizam Shahi.

'I know. I think, I should send crown prince Ibrahim to suppress the rebels.'

Ibrahim failed to supress the rebellion and the rebels marched to the city to depose Burhan. Despite his feeble health, Burhan rode out against the rebels and defeated them. But the exertion of the campaign proved too much for him and he died soon after.

Ibrahim succeeded his father but failed to control the ever growing influence of nobles, notably of Miyan Manjhu Deccani, the chief minister. After four months, in a battle with Bijapur, which was ensued purely by a clash of the personal ambitions of Ahmednagar nobles, Ibrahim lost his life.

'Ibrahim's infant son, Bahadur, will be the new sultan.' Chand Bibi announced, pressing claim for her nephew's son.

'No. There is a mature legal heir, the twelve-year-old Ahmad in Daulatabad,' Miyan Manjhu opposed.

A stunned Chand Bibi tried to get the support of Abyssinian nobles to suppress the internal trouble and also to strengthen the claim for Bahadur's ascension to the throne. But, Miyan Manjhu outsmarted her and won over Abyssinians as well as other nobles. Thus, Ahmad became the king, and Bahadur was imprisoned. However, Chand Bibi was quick to expose the lineage fraud of Ahmad and succeeded in convincing the nobles that Ahmad was not a true royal blood prince. She, thus, reclaimed the throne for Bahadur. But, another faction of nobles presented another contender, Moti Shah, a bazaar boy, and proclaimed him as king.

A frustrated Miyan Manjhu was now distressed; he thought that the only way to win back his power was to invite the Mughals camping in Malwa. He sent a letter to Prince Murad, son of Emperor Akbar, explaining the vulnerable politics of Ahmednagar and invited him to annex the Sultanate.

Fortunately for Ahmednagar, before the letters could reach Prince Murad, nobles of her opposite camp fell out amongst themselves regarding distribution of office. Chand Bibi watched the situation carefully and soon called for Miyan Manjhu.

'Bibi, I bitterly repent my folly of having invited the Mughals.' Miyan Manjhu cut himself a sorry figure.

'It's always better to accept a mistake.' Chand Bibi consoled him.'Miyan Manjhu, now you should plan to resist the enemy. I will unite the nobles.'

'Bibi, I don't have the courage to plan. I feel like a straw before the storm. I see ghosts of the enemy everywhere.'

'Miyan, muster all your courage and fight for Ahmednagar,' Chand Bibi commanded.

'I know Bibi, you want me die,' he uttered, voice broken.

'If you can't fight the Mughals, then convene a meeting of nobles. Call everyone—the Abyssinians, Deccanies, foreigners…everyone.'

He convened the meeting, but he could not bear the strain of the huge distrust among the nobles.

Shrewdly, he announced in the meeting, 'Nizam Shahi has been our ruler since generations and Chand Bibi is the guardian of Nizam Shahi. Only she can solicit assistance from Bijapur and Golkunda. I propose to leave all the affairs of the state in her hands.'

But, despite assurances from Chand Bibi Miyan Manjhu was never sure how Ahmednagar would take on the mighty Mughals. Therefore, he did not stay back to fight the Mughals. Instead, he fled leaving the responsibility of protecting the honour and dignity of Ahmednagar on Chand Bibi's shoulders.

I need to put the prevailing confusion to rest, thought Chand Bibi as she formed a composite council of action consisting of nobles from all factions. She, then, appointed a wakil of her choice and proclaimed young Bahadur Nizam Shah as the sovereign of Ahmednagar.

'Prince Murad is accompanied by the famous poet and Mughal commander Rahim Khan Khanan and Raja Ali Khan, the ruler of Khandesh. They have camped near the northern gate. When a few shots were exchanged,the Mughals retreated tactically. Now, I hear that Murad endeavours to win popular support for his enterprise,' the new wakil Muhammad Khan informed the regent.

'He must be telling the people that he would safeguard their lives and protect them from the high-handedness of our nobles,' Chand Bibi guessed, as public suffering due to internal skirmishes of the nobles was no secret.

'Yes, Bibi. The Mughals have also marked the ground for trenches against the fort.'

Chand Bibi thought for a moment and then said, 'Let Shamshir Khan and Mir Muhammad Jaman attack the Mughal and break their ranks and file.'

Chand Bibi's daring suggestion stunned everyone. Launching a surprise attack outside the fort with a couple of platoons on a huge army like that of the mighty Mughals was a suicidal idea. Everyone opposed it, but she remained unmoved. Next morning, the sudden attack of the two commanders of Ahmednagar broke the Mughal ranks and forced them to retreat. Prince Murad decided to lift the siege of the fort.

'Let our victories be made known to people,' Chand Bibi announced. 'I also want the cruelty unleashed by the Mughal generals on the inhabitants of Burhanabad be known to everyone.'

Following his father's policy of not troubling the civilian populace, Murad had instructed his generals accordingly. But when the seige went longer, impatient soldiers began looting local villagers. Prince Murad was enraged by the cruelty of his troops. He even ordered public execution of the miscreants. By then, the people no longer relied upon the Mughal prince's assurance of good governance.

Unfortunately, even this temporary victory of Ahmednagar

provided to its amirs an opportunity to pursue their own individual ambitions. Though the Mughals were not far away, few of the Ahmednagar nobles, under Ikhlas Khan, hastened to Daulatabad. There they declared their independence from Bahadur Shah and proclaimed a new boy as the new king of Ahmednagar. From there, with 12,000 riders, these rebels advanced towards Ahmednagar with the objective of wrestling power out of the hands of Chand Bibi.

In an another act of rebellion, a second faction of nobles under Abhang Khan went to Bid where the amirs raised a canopy over his head and declared him as the sultan of Ahmednagar.

'Send an envoy to Miyan Manjhu. Tell him that we can settle our scores later. Urge him to go to Bijapur and solicit assistance,' Chand Bibi asked her wakil.

'Ikhlas Khan has rebelled and he is marching towards us with his 12,000 men.'

'Send spies to the Mughals and spread the rumour that our contingent of 12,000 will attack them near Paithan on the banks of Godavari,' Chand Bibi told a baffled Muhammad Khan.

That was brilliant move on Bibi's part, because the ruse worked in their favour. After getting the information, the Mughals interrupted the progress of the rebels and inflicted a crushing defeat on them.

But, Chand Bibi understood it was just a temporary relief.

'Wakil Sahib, send a confidential message to Abhang Khan. Convince him to come to talking terms with Miyan Manjhu. Then, both of them should march to Daulatabad and expel the Mughals. I will send 500 Abyssinians to assist them.'

Muhammad Khan looked at his regent in disbelief. 'How

is it possible to ask two opponents to join hands?'But, Chand Bibi was determined.

The last week of December 1595 was very cold. Very early in the morning, Prince Murad, in the company of his generals, inspected the surroundings of the fort and marked out the ground for the trenches and distributed commands and gave them specific instructions.

Despite the Mughal siege of the fort, Abhang Khan, the leader of the Ahmednagar rebels, attacked the Mughals and blocked their way into the fort. But the Mughals quickly responded and the entire army of Abhang Khan was largely diminished.

'Let us surround the fort from all sides. Men must move forward quickly and in all directions in the trenches,' an angry Murad commanded his men during the fight.

'Look at Murad. I have never seen him spending all this time with his men,' Raja Ali Khan said admiringly.

'Yes, he is engaged with the soldiers in carrying forward the trenches, in filling the ditch, and in erecting batteries overlooking the wall of the fort,' even the worst critic of Murad, Rahim Khan Khanan agreed.

'This will be an easy win,' Ali Khan was saying when the Ahmednagar sentries deployed on the gates attacked the Mughal engineers and soldiers. Throughout the day, such attacks continued and rendered all the Mughal progress useless.

'I told you, it is not easy,' Khan Khanan chuckled.

'Rahim, I hear that Chand Bibi herself is supervising the defences of the fort and affairs of the army.'

'I am told that she has not rested for a moment and has

guided her workers and soldiers with a great insight. They have become a united force.'

'But how long will they last against the huge Mughal army?'

'Raja Ali Khan, rivalry and jealousy are not alien to us either. If we lose the momentum, the Ahmednagar garrison will get time to put their defences in order and may also get support from other Deccan states,' Rahim Khan Khanan opined.

An experienced campaigner, Rahim was not off the mark. On Chand Bibi's initiative, the local Koli tribes and Miyan Manjhu had opened a surprise attack on the Mughals and also intercepted their communication and supply lines. Chand Bibi had also dispatched her envoys to organize a grand coalition of Bijapur, Golkunda and the Nizam Shahi's armies. On the other hand, Murad's problems were aggravated by the scarcity of provisions and the hostility between his commanders.

In Ahmednagar, Chand Bibi succeeded in bringing Ikhlas Khan and Miyan Manjhu together, and Bijapur and Golkunda agreed to send 70,000 troops without delay.

'Shahjada Huzur, I am certain that Raja Ali Khan helped in restoring communication between garrison and the outside world. He also helped Ahmednagar in getting smuggled arms and provisions,' a Mughal spy informed Murad.

Prince Murad fumed, 'Let's launch an attack on the fort. And see to it that Raja Ali Khan be discharged from all war related duties.'

Raja Ali Khan heard about the Prince's announcement and decided to save the situation by writing a letter to Chand Bibi.

'Sultana Sahiba, I know your situation. Your reputation and hundreds of lives can be saved if you surrender the fort to the prince and take in lieu thereof any other fort of your choice.'

'Why would Raja Ali Khan propose something like this?' Chand Bibi consulted her amirs.

When the amirs could not agree to a unanimous reply, Chand Bibi decided to send a firm reply by rejecting the proposal.

The Mughals replied by carrying five mines under the bastions on one side of the fort. Murad ordered to fill them with gunpowder.

'Tomorrow morning, the mines will explode and we will take the fort,' the Mughals celebrated prematurely.

Chand Bibi's spies told her about the mines. She quickly gathered her men and inspired them to sacrifice their lives for the cause of the kingdom. As a result, in the middle of the night hundreds of people climbed down the fort, discovered the mines, removed the gunpowder and filled them with stone and earth. Before dawn, they had rendered four mines useless.

Next morning, when the Mughal army assembled to set fire to the mines, only one exploded, blowing about fifty yards of the fort wall, but no other mine exploded.

'Before the Mughals attack, let us repair the breach,' Chand Bibi put all the masons on wall repair work and ordered soldiers to shoot at the enemy from the fort walls.

Clad in glittering armour, mounted on an elephant, when she stood at the forefront, the soldiers let loose a volley of arrows, grenades and shots at the enemy.

'Martyrdom is certain if the enemy's wound kills me, so why should I hide in the palace? Let us fight and win. If it happens otherwise, I have brought a chalice of poison to save myself from the indignity of falling into enemy hands.'

The Mughals started retaliating. Their booming guns were emitting fire. But, the undaunted Chand Bibi was leading from the front. The Mughal army made desperate efforts to enter the fort but they were beaten back.

This accomplishment infused a new confidence in the people of the garrison. Thousands of hands came forward to work ceaselessly to defend the fort. Chand Bibi remained present on the spot—cheering and inspiring her people. People responded with the chant, 'Chand Sultana...Chand Sultana.'

Defeated, disappointed and distraught, Prince Murad spent the whole night counselling his generals. Khan Khanan was still not cooperating. Murad decided to lead from the front.

He advanced to the breached wall and dismounted from his horse at the very edge of the moat, to address his troops.

'Brave soldiers, serve the Mughals loyally and break the back of Ahmednagar. I promise each one of you 100 gold coins and a promotion in rank.'

The Mughal army attacked the fort with a new zeal. Murad reinforced the attack with his Ahadi troops. The Ahadis were battle-worthy and the toughest fighters. They delivered the most vigorous attack on the fort.

Chand Sultana, standing at a fort canopy, directed her defenders. Bolstered by the success of last evening, they showered fire on the Mughal army. The battle went on from sunrise to sunset; the Mughals showed the greatest valour but Chand Sultana's defence was like an iron wall. After heavy causalities in his army, a disgusted Murad withdrew his force.

'Prince Murad, the soldiers are tired and exhausted. We are short of provisions and combined armies of Bijapur and Golkunda are approaching faster,' a spy reported.

Murad looked at Rahim Khan Khanan in disgust but could not do much more. Rahim was a favourite of his father.

'Rahim, my worry is that once the joint Deccan force comes here, Chand Bibi will meekly surrender to them. The better course is to begin negotiations.'

'Who will negotiate from our side?' Rahim asked.

'You,' replied Murad with straight face. 'Ask them to give us Berar and Daulatabad.'

Discussions went on for a long time as Chand Bibi did not agree to give up Daulatabad. She was also worried as she could not trust her ever-scheming nobles within the volatile Deccan politics. Both the sides were hard pressed and agreed that the Mughals would get Berar and retreat from Ahmednagar.

That was Chand Bibi's biggest accomplishment. She had forced the mighty Mughals to retreat.

Unfortunately, the Ahmednagar politics returned to its internal feuds immediately after the enemy withdrew. Different fractions claimed the throne for their protégés. Miyan Manjhu, Abhang Khan and others came out in open rebellion. In such a situation, Chand Bibi sought help from her nephew's son, the Sultan of Bijapur, to crush the rebellion.

When Miyan Manjhu heard about it, he sought an audience with the regent and apologized.

'Miyan Manjhu, you have no friends left here. If Bahadur turns his back, you will not have any in Bijapur either. I suggest you leave Ahmednagar and retire to Bijapur.'

She thereby successfully thwarted the ambitious plans of the nobles and restored peace in Ahmednagar after many years of chaos. The Nizam Shahi forces also defeated the Mughals in the battle of Asthi, with the help of the Deccan alliance.

Peaceful life in Ahmednagar continued until 1598, when the Uzbek king Abdullah Khan died. His death gave Emperor Akbar an opportunity to turn his attention to the Deccan problem. Khan Khanan had been recalled and Abul Fazl was sent in his place to help Murad. But the humiliation of defeat from Chand Bibi had led Prince Murad to excessive drinking. As a result, he suffered from epilepsy and chronic dyspepsia.

A worried Akbar asked him to return to Agra. But, unable to bear his disgraceful recall, despite his serious illness, Murad set out to win Ahmednagar. When Abhang Khan in Ahmednagar heard it, he once again raised the flag of rebellion. Chand Bibi was restricted to the fort. However, Prince Murad died on the way in 1599.

An angry Akbar decided to march in person to Ahmednagar. He won Burhanpur and then opened the siege of Asirgarh. The expedition was taking time and he commanded his son Daniyal and Khan Khanan to march quickly to Ahmednagar.

Upon the approach of Prince Daniyal and with the possibility of him being unable to resist the Mughals, Abhang Khan expressed his desire to come into terms with Chand Bibi. But she refused to listen to his gambits and in sheer frustration, Abhang Khan fled from Ahmednagar.

'Sultana, the Mughals have sieged the fort and commenced mining the walls,' her courtier Hamid Khan, a eunuch, told Chand Bibi.

She already knew it.

'Hamid, we cannot withstand the Mughal onslaught again, particularly when the Mughal Emperor himself is within a short distance. We will continue fighting the invaders,'

Chand Bibi declared and started preparing for war against the mightiest empire of the world.

The siege dragged on for many months. It created panic in the garrison when there was no provision and ammunition left.

'We should fight and defend the fort till our last breath,' Hamid Khan suggested.

Chand Bibi looked at her people crying and dying with hunger.

'No, for me, the life and the property of my people are paramount. Hamid, I am ready to surrender the fort, if the Mughals guarantee safety to them.'

Hamid Khan looked at her in disagreement and ran into the streets.

'Chand Bibi is a traitor! Chand Bibi is a traitor! She is in league with the Mughals.'

'No it cannot be!' No one believed the eunuch.

'I heard it from her. Akbar will add her to his harem and she would be his favourite sultana.' The eunuch did not stop there but went on spreading malicious and false rumours.

Soon, the people started believing the eunuch and were filled with anger. The excited mob headed by her rushed into Chand Bibi's private chamber and put her to death.

The tragic ending filled Mary Palmer's eyes with tears. She looked at her husband, who was listening with his head down.

'Philip, if the Britons are proud of their queens, and the people of Delhi of their Raziya, the Deccanies could justifiably be proud of their Chand Bibi.'

She began sobbing and continued.

'Philip, my grandfather used to say that, so great was the love she inspired, that the peasants of the Western hills refused for many years to believe that she was dead. She had escaped, they said, through an underground passage and is hiding in some deep fold of the Sahyadri mountains. When the time will come, she would again reveal herself and drive out the Mughals across the Vindhyas and bring back the golden years of Ahmednagar.'

Abbakka

Before climbing those unending stairs of the majestic Safavid Palace, Pietro Della Valle looked at its grand dome shining against the sky. The distinctive bulbous vault decorated with colour-glazed tiles and a complex vegetal pattern was visible to him in its entirety. The crown of the dome was nearly piercing into the heart of the heaven.

'Indeed, only the Safavids and the Mughals can prick the canvas of the blue sky like this.'

Pietro was about to meet the Great Shah Abbas, who was then presiding over the Persian Empire. Standing tall on shoulders of the Armenian expertise of silk and its trade networks, Shah Abbas had put Persia at the zenith of prosperity.

A common enemy, the Ottomans had traumatized both the Persians and the Europeans for centuries. Hatred for the Ottomans had made Shah Abbas highly tolerant towards the Christians. In fact, once he had famously declared that he preferred the dust from the shoes of the lowest Christian to the highest Ottoman personage. Pietro was well aware of the tragic shipwreck of a Safavid diplomatic mission to Europe, on its way back to Persia. Apart from meeting many European kings, the mission also had a long audience with Pope Clement

VIII at Rome, and this cultural mission had left the Europeans fascinated about Persia and its culture.

Contrary to Pietro's expectations, Shah quickly put his Italian guest at ease. Pietro's charming style of narration of the who's who in Europe and other unknown societies around the world had impressed the Shah. The Shah, on his part, had kind words to say about everyone except his three sworn enemies, the Ottomans, the Spanish and the Portuguese.

'Pietro, I like the way the English do business. But not the Portuguese,' Shah complained.

'Few decades ago, the Portuguese established their base in Persian Gulf that I had overlooked. I thought they were doing business like the other Europeans do, but when they began fortification of Bahrain and converting the Shias to Christianity, I sensed an alarm. I sent a small army under Imam Quli Khan Undiladze ordering their expulsion from Persia. It was tough but the English ships helped me. Despite that, those wretched Portuguese captured Hormuz and declared it as their colony. I had to kill all of them to declare Hormuz a free trade centre.'

'Oh, then they moved to Goa?' Pietro asked.

'No. They were there before the Mughals had arrived in India.' Picking a fresh glass of wine, Shah lamented, 'and Jahangir is doing nothing. Despite my warning, he had not thrown the Portuguese out of Goa. Except Abbakka, no Indian ruler had the heart to fight the Portuguese.'

Pietro had never heard that name before. 'Who is he?'

'He?' Shah looked questioningly at Pietro. 'You don't know about Abbakka?'

'Pietro, Hindustan does not mean only Dilli or Agra. It is

a land made up of hundreds of states. Abbakka was a queen of a small principality in Hindustan.'

'A queen?'

'Yes, a queen!' Pietro wondered that the great Shah of Persia was now telling him about a woman ruler whom he had never heard of before.

'Ullal is a small coastal town nestled in a strip of land between the Western Ghat Hills and the Arabian Sea. The western coastline region between south of Goa and north of Kozhikode is referred to as Tulu Nadu. It is a fertile land that gets plenty of rain from the southwestern monsoons. Surrounded by thick rain forests, the villages and the towns along the shoreline are natural harbours and ports. The people of Tulu Nadu had established trade routes with the Arabs as early as in seventh century and benefitted from the flourishing maritime trade of pepper and ginger with the west.'

'Your Majesty, then why is the king of Portugal called the "Grocer King" instead of the Arabs?' Pietro could not resist his query.

'True,' the Shah said patiently. 'In the year 1498, a Portuguese named Vasco de Gama landed in the town of Kozhikode. In the ensuing years, the Portuguese consolidated their power and made Goa their colony and they intended to control the trade between Europe and India. Therefore, they want to control all the harbours and ports. Their full control over the Arabian Sea ensures that all vessels coming to the western shores of Hindustan have to navigate through the blockade of the Portuguese naval armada. The Portuguese are largely successful in this.

'Indian spices, cloth, rice, medicines, jaggery and sugar

are in great demand in Europe and Mediterranean countries. John III was a shrewd king and wanted to have a monopoly over the spice trade. The success of the Portuguese oriental trade earned John III the title of the "Grocer King". During his reign, the Portuguese became the first Europeans to make contact with both Japan and China. But, it was Hindustan that touched the heart of John III. For his profitable Hindustani trade, he had willingly abandoned the Islamic territories in North Africa.

'However, minor settlements along the coast such as Ullal did not obey the Portuguese. In John III's life time, the Portuguese launched three major offensives on Mangalore and Ullal, but failed to crush them.'

It was unthinkable for Pietro that a small principality led by a woman defeated the might of John III, the shining star of the Portuguese House of Aviz.

Shah Abbas smiled. 'Ullal is a unique port in south of the confluence of two rivers, Netravathi and Gurupura. Ullal, Someshwara and Mangalore were three important townships in Tulu Nadu, which the Portuguese were eyeing.'

'Someshwara sounds like a religious place.' Pietro made an observation.

'Yes, very much.' Shah paused and then asked, 'Pietro, the Ottoman Turks fight with us. You know why?'

'You are a Shia and they are Turks.'

'True. But the Hindustanis are different. The Abbakkas are Jains. Yet, they have built a beautiful temple dedicated to a Hindu god, Shiva, and their family deity is Somnatheshwara.'

Looking at his astonished Italian guest, Shah Abbas laughed.

'The Abbakkas belong to the Chowta clan. The Chowtas were Rajputs of Gujarat. They had built the famous Somnath Temple, which was later plundered by Mehmud Gaznavi. The Waghelas drove the Chowtas out of Saurashtra and later became subordinates to the great Vijayanagar Empire and ruled from the temple town of Moodabidri.'

Shah Abbas was enjoying the dialogue and continued, 'Pietro, in the year 1525 when the Portuguese attacked South Kanara Coast and destroyed Mangalore, Abbakka was the queen of Ullal. In 1570, when Kozhikode and Ullal defeated the Portuguese, Abbakka was still the queen. And she still rules Ullal.'

'Your Majesty, is she immortal?'

'That's why I address her only in plural. Many societies like Chowta in Tulu Nadu are matrilineal, where a daughter inherits property from her mother. There are two or more Abbakkas. Here, I am talking about Queen Abbakka II.'

During the reign of Hiriya Abbakka, mother of Queen Abbakka II, the Portuguese first attacked South Kanara Coast and destroyed Mangalore. The Portuguese stationed an armed garrison after fortifying Mangalore and enmeshed Ullal within the web of colonization and commercial exploitation. This alerted Hiriya Abbakka and she started preparing for a possible future conflict with the Portuguese who had started demanding favours and discounts in trade and export taxes.

An influential royal, Thirumala Raya assisted Hiriya Abbakka's efforts enthusiastically and worked hard to make Ullal militarily strong. He also groomed Abbakka II to take up future responsibilities of Ullal. She learnt the art of diplomacy from the wise ministers, and martial arts from the best trainers of Vijayanagar.

Thirumala Raya astutely arranged an alliance of marriage between a young Abbakka and handsome Lakshmappa Arasa, the Banga prince of Bangadi. Banga was a powerful dynasty of Mangalore. This alliance strengthened the position of Ullal and irked the Portuguese.

On her deathbed, Hiriya Abbakka called her daughter, 'Abbakka, when the Portuguese warships were heading for Mangalore, I suggested carrying the war into the enemy's camp. My ministers were against it. I was sure that once they made Mangalore their headquarters, the Portuguese would attack us.

Therefore, ignoring the advice of my ministers, I sailed to Mangalore. We set ablaze the fourteen Portuguese ships anchored there, with our fire-tipped arrows. We assumed that they would take years to recover but in no time they received reinforcement from Goa. Their counter attack resulted in our humiliating defeat.'

Queen Mother Abbakka sighed heavily. Before breathing her last, she said, 'Child, that humiliation still irks my heart and I am carrying that burden.'

'Mother, don't grieve. I promise to avenge our humiliation.'

Before she could hear her daughter's promise, Hiriya Abbakka died repenting her defeat in the hands of the Portuguese.

Next day, Abbakka was crowned as the new queen of Ullal. She was fiercely independent, full of purpose and determination. She refused to bargain with the Portuguese and prevented them from having any foothold in the region.

She revamped the port of Ullal for exports and expanded it. She trained her people in making Ullal stronger and to oppose any Portuguese advances. Very soon, she became a symbol of the patriotic fervour among her subjects.

Abbakka also sought assistance from her husband, now the king of Bangadi and Mangalore.

'I am thinking of stopping the favours to the Portuguese and not selling spices and cloth to them.'

'Don't be so naïve. Remember what happened to your mother.' Lakshmappa was pro-Portuguese and feared their wrath. Their marriage was more of convenience than conviction.

'I remember what happened to my mother.' Abbakka replied back, 'that's why I am determined to drive them out of our land.'

'In that case, you fight them if they attack Ullal.' Lakshmappa retorted rudely.

'Please try to understand.' Abbakka tried to reason with him. 'The Portuguese fort in Mangalore is on your land. They can use it to attack Ullal any time. Why don't you make them quit your fort?'

'Abbakka, I am not stupid like you. I know my limitations and also the might of the Portuguese.'

'Lakshmappa, then you go your way; I am not afraid of the Portuguese.'

That was the beginning of an open discontent between the couple.

When her husband refused to assist her, Abbakka gained support from the powerful King Venkatappanayaka of Bidnur and began to forge alliance with other local chiefs as well. The fearless Queen's efforts began to rattle the Portuguese dream of controlling the maritime trade.

'Buca Devi Chowta has become a major threat to us. Chiefs of the western coast are inclining to support her. A sense of daring among coastal Indians is evident. Lord, if we don't take immediate steps to curb this rebellion, our dream will never be realized,' Antonio Noronha, a powerful noble urged John III in Lisbon's royal court.

'They call her The Fearless. She promptly rejects our demands of payment of tribute as she knows that any such payment will be construed as her succumbing to the Portuguese authority.' Dom Alvaro de Silveira, an admiral in the Portuguese navy, seconded Noronha.

'Then what are you waiting for? Go and teach her a lesson.' John III shouted at them.

Humiliated in the court, Admiral Silveira quickly returned to Goa to plan an end to Abbakka's exploits.

Admiral Silveira decided that what could not be won on the battlefield could be won by deceit and larceny. His envoy warned Lakshmappa to not send any reinforcement to Ullal under the threat of burning Mangalore. Lakshmappa himself was looking for an opportunity to humiliate his wife. As per the matrilineal custom among the Chowtas, all three children of Abbakka and Lakshmappa were in her custody and were living in Ullal. Their eldest daughter was now of marriageable age.

One day, when Lakshmappa visited Ullal, their daughter wished to visit Aadhishwara Parshvanatha Basadi temple in Mangalore. 'No, the temple is very close to the Portuguese Fort.' Abbakka refused permission.

'So what? Mangalore belongs to my father and the Portuguese are his friends,' their daughter countered.

'Child, but they are not my friends.'

'Mother, are you afraid of the Portuguese?'

This childish stubbornness irked Abbakka. 'I am not afraid of the Portuguese. If you wish, you may visit the temple.'

When the princess went out after having got her way, Abbakka shared her worries with Lakshmappa.

'Lakshmappa, I am worried for her. We should find her a good match.'

'I know one,' Lakshmappa grinned.

'Who?'

'My nephew, Kamaraya. He will succeed me as the king of Bangadi.'

The proposal stunned Abbakka. 'No. My daughter shall not marry him. I will find her a valorous, kind-hearted man of character.'

Her refusal made Lakshmappa extremely angry. 'Abbakka, you have insulted my clan. Hereafter I will never step in your kingdom.' Abusing his wife, Lakshmappa stomped out of her palace.

An angry and humiliated Lakshmappa quickly hatched a conspiracy.

Unaware of her father's intentions, the princess left Ullal for Mangalore the next morning.

The moment the princess came out of the temple, Lakshmappa's men kidnapped her and killed her escorts. But the Queen had a premonition that the Portuguese might create trouble for the princess; therefore, she had sent a platoon after her. The soldiers from Ullal attacked the kidnappers and overpowered them in no time.

This incident horrified the Queen and she lost no time

in finding a suitable groom for her daughter and quickly got her married.

The kidnapping attempt created a huge chasm between the couple and Lakshmappa never visited Ullal again.

Soon after this incident, Admiral Silveira attacked Ullal. After a daylong battle, there was no clear winner. An uneasy truce was declared; the unhappy Portuguese authorities replaced Admiral Silveira with a younger Louis De' Mellow.

Abbakka began restoration of the ruined fort of Ullal and building bigger and better merchant ships for trade with distant countries. She often visited the temple of Goddess Durga at Polali. During one such visit, Lakshmappa's men attacked her. They asked her to step down from her palanquin. When she refused, they used force and killed her escorts. Forcefully, she was taken to Lakshmappa.

Lakshmappa forcibly paraded her before his men. But, Abbakka turned the show around when in the middle of the huge crowd, she challenged his wisdom.

'Deva, a word from you would have brought me here. Why did you choose to send armed men instead? Did the Portuguese ask you to kidnap me? How can you betray and humiliate your own wife?'

The murmuring among the people became loud and widespread. Abbakka challenged her husband, 'Deva, I must get back to Ullal to perform my rightful duty. You dare not stop me.'

A frustrated Lakshmappa shouted at his soldiers, 'Stop her, stop her!' But no one moved.

Meanwhile, De' Mellow secretly recruited Lakshamappa's nephew Kamaraya to plot against his uncle and usurp the throne of Manga. The conspiracy led by his nephew and the humiliation in front of his own people following Abbakka's abduction never allowed Lakshmappa to recover and he died soon after. Kamaraya became the king of Bangadi in 1556.

Two years later, Louis De' Mellow assembled a huge Portuguese army and attacked Ullal. They ransacked and torched the town down. In retaliation, the people of Ullal, the fishing community of Mogaveeras, the Moplah Mussalmans, backward castes like the Bilavas and many others joined hands and attacked the Portuguese with weapons provided by the Queen. Their attack was too robust for the Portuguese to withstand.

This victory bolstered the prestige of the Queen in the entire west coast and abroad. Many local chiefs offered her help. Many influential kings such as the Zamorin of Kozhikode offered her a partnership in export trade.

The Queen promptly picked up the proposal. Soon, joint fleets filled with loads of mercantile goods of Ullal and Kozhikode began sailing in the Arabian Sea. The alarmed Portuguese sent their envoy to Mangalore to lodge a protest and warn the Queen.

'Our governor warns you that any direct trade with the non-Portuguese will be treated as an act of hostility.'

'Is that all?' The Queen retorted.

'No. His Highness reminds you that the annual tribute from your state is long overdue.'

'Are you finished? Kindly tell your governor that Ullal is a sovereign state and does not take orders from Portugal. I refuse to pay any tribute to Portugal.'

'You will repent it, your Highness.' The envoy threatened

before marching off.

The Portuguese were now alarmed at the pace of expanded trade at the port of Ullal. They again resorted to harassing tactics which could not deter the Queen. In frustration, the Portuguese perpetrated wanton destruction on Mangalore; countless men, women and children were put to death. The Portuguese army also plundered temples, burnt ships and finally set the city on fire.

On the diplomatic front, the Portuguese governor passed a series of edicts against Ullal. He called Abbakka's alliance with the Zamorin of Kozhikode illegal and her trade with Persia and Arabia an unfriendly act. Abbakka dismissed these rulings with contempt and scorn.

The Portuguese were further infuriated with the non-conformist behaviour of Abbakka. They were more alarmed by the maturing diplomatic relations between her and the king of Keladi, and with the Zamorin of Kozhikode. Ignoring the warnings of the Portuguese, Abbakka continued exporting spices and other goods to the Middle East with the Zamorin's help. Once, when the Portuguese captured a Ullal merchant ship in mid-sea, an infuriated Abbakka attacked the Mangalore Fort and destroyed a Portuguese factory there.

This retaliatory attack by the Queen shook the Portuguese's roots in India. King Sebastian I sent a stern message to the Portuguese viceroy in India, Antonio Noronha. Antonio chose one of his ablest general, Joao Peixoto, to crush the rebellion.

Never inhistory had such a huge enemy force been seen in Ullal. Charging like an enraged bull, General Peixoto's army captured the city and entered the royal court. This sudden attack left Ullal defenceless. Abbakka managed to escape with the help of a few local Mussalmans, and took refuge in a mosque.

When Abbakka reached the mosque, the local qazi and all the other prominent Moplahs volunteered to fight for her. With the help of the Moplahs, she could assemble around 200 fighters.

She mounted an attack on the Portuguese. General Peixoto was not expecting a counter attack so soon. The moment he heard the noise outside the court, he quickly gathered his soldiers. The Queen attacked like a hurricane and no enemy could stand before her. In the battle that ensued, General Peixoto was killed along with 70 Portuguese soldiers. Some Portuguese soldiers were taken prisoners and many of them fled. Hearing the news of the battle, people from the neighbourhood flocked to Ullal and joined the Queen's army.

The shame of this defeat numbed both Admiral Mascarenhas at the Mangalore Fort and Viceroy Noronho in Goa. Noronha quickly sent reinforcement to Mangalore but before they could reach, Abbakka and her soldiers had already attacked the Mangalore Fort. Admiral Mascarenhas was killed in the fight and the Portuguese were forced to evacuate the Mangalore Fort.

A humiliated Noronha marched south with 3,000 men and several battleships. The surprise pre-dawn attack caught Abbakka off guard—she was returning from Somanatheshwara after offering her prayers. Without wasting time, she donned her battle armour and mounted on her horse to fight the invaders. She challenged her men and inspired them to defeat the attackers.

'Let us push them back to the sea. Let us fight them on

land and the sea, on the streets and the beaches.'

She launched a fierce counter offensive. Unfortunately, she was wounded in a barrage of gunfire and was whisked away by her loyal soldiers to a secluded place. The Portuguese searched in vain for the wounded Queen. Few say that she was caught later, while few say that she remained free. But Pietro, until the end, she kept encouraging her soldiers and urged them to never give up in their fight for their motherland.

Pietro remained silent for a long time. Torches were now lit inside the palace. It was time to go. Pietro stood up and took permission to leave.

'If you plan to go to India, then you must visit Ullal and meet the Queen. She is a lioness among humans.' Shah Abbas bid adieu to the traveller.

Few years later, Pietro Della Valle arrived at Ullal in 1624 and enquired about the Queen. Abbakka was still the ruler.

'Sister, daughter or grand-daughter?' Pietro was not sure and nobody came forward to explain.

'How can I meet her?' he asked a shopkeeper.

'You need not to find her. She will find you.' The old shopkeeper laughed showing his toothless grin.

'But when?'

The shopkeeper smiled but said nothing.

One day, he saw a woman walking barefoot in the middle of the marching soldiers. 'It's the Queen …the Queen,' his guide whispered. A servant was holding a palm leaf umbrella over a slightly plump lady's head as protection from the sun. The lady had dark complexion and was clad in an ordinary cotton sari with another cloth covering her head and upper body.

'She looks like a kitchen-woman or a laundress, rather than a delicate and noble Queen,' a disappointed Pietro uttered.

'She is the queen,' his guide almost pushed him towards her.

'Move … move.' The Queen's escorts gently whisked him to stay away.

Pietro went closer instead and greeted her. She was Abbakka. Pietro introduced himself as a non-Portuguese European, and told her that he had come from the land of the Pope.

'I have seen several countries, your Majesty. And have had the privilege of meeting the Persian and the Mughal emperors.' The Queen smiled, 'After seeing the great Persian and Mughal kings, what is there to see in this wilderness?'

'I came only to see you, your Majesty. You are so well-known in my part of the world.'

The Queen laughed. Her teeth were like pearls and her smile flashed like diamonds in a dark night.

The Queen made arrangements for Pietro's stay. Pietro remained in Ullal for many weeks. However, the Queen never shared her or her mother's eulogies with him. With motherly concern, she enquired about his health and sent nurses to take care of him when he fell ill.

Much later, Pietro Della Valle wrote,

> *She is a noble queen who loved her subjects, personally supervised welfare measures and settled disputes in the evenings. I wondered if this was the woman who was eulogised and made a cult figure all over Europe overnight for having made Portugal bite the dust by*

decimating its troops with a vengeance. Whatever her appearance, she was all dignity and aplomb in her bearing. Her words were soft and balmy. It looked as though she had a clear-cut vision and a well-defined purpose. And I feel the way she covered her face at times during interlocution represented the politeness and geniality of the Orientals.... Her sober and nonchalant elegance has earned her the nick name of being the 'tough woman'.

Chennamma of Keladi

The Mughal Emperor Aurangzeb ordered for the drums to be beaten to celebrate the death of Shivaji, his chief foe who had been resisting his Deccan dream for so long. However, his joy proved to be short lived. The relentless Marathas, under Shivaji's son Shambhuji, continued attacking the Mughal dominion.

Aurangzeb's wrath against Shambhuji was already fuelled—he had anticipated that Shambhuji who had spent many years as a political hostage of the Mughals and also served as a mansabdar in the Mughal court would be more amicable towards him than his father. But, Shambhuji's attack on Bahadurkhan Kokaltash, a trusted relative of the Emperor, and his act of providing shelter to Aurangzeb's rebel son Sultan Muhammad Akbar convinced the Emperor that the new chhatrapati could not be trusted either.

Aurangzeb decided to teach Shambhuji a lesson and marched towards the Maratha stronghold with half a million troops and 40,000 animals.

Shambhuji was captured in February 1689 at Sangameshwar. He was brutally tortured and later beheaded with an axe at Talpur, near Pune. His brutal end put the Maratha confederacy into disarray. In such a crisis, Shambhaji's half-brother Rajaram assumed the throne as the third chhatrapati. Before he could settle down in his seat, the Mughals knocked at the doors of the Raigad fort, the seat of Chhatrapati.

'The Mughals have sieged Raigad. Jinji remains our only hope. You go there and consolidate the Maratha position,' Queen Tara Bai advised her husband Rajaram to leave the fort quickly.

'How can I reach Jinji? No king will help me and make enemies out of the Mughals,' Rajaram was shaky.

'I know a queen who can help you.'

'A queen! Against Aurangzeb?'

'Yes. Queen Chennamma of Keladi. She will help you reach Jinji,' Tara Bai was very sure.

'I see the merit in the Queen's suggestion,' Amatya Ramchandra Pant seconded her. Even Yesubai, Shambhuji's wife approved the idea.

'How can I trust an unknown queen?'

'Once you know about her, you will trust.'

Keladi is a kingdom in the Malenadu area of Karnataka. It covers the western and eastern slopes of the Western Ghats or the Shahyadri mountain range, roughly 60 miles in width. The hills of Malenadu are thickly forested.

'A great warrior, Chowdappa Nayaka founded the Keladi kingdom in 1499 AD. The Keladi Nayakas of Ikkeri and their descendants are known as Muddurajas or Mudiraj and they belong to the Bedar or Valmiki community,' Tara Bai went on about the royals of Keladi.

'In about 1645, Shivappa Nayaka, considered to be the greatest amongst the Keladi kings, ascended the throne. Known for his just rule and administrative reforms, Shivappa Nayaka systematized the governance and the collection of taxes in such a way that people called him, "Shistina Shivappa Nayaka".'

'What is that?' Rajaram enquired.

'That means Shivappa Nayaka, the Facilitator of Discipline and Order,' Tara Bai explained.

Shivappa Nayaka's son Somashekhara Nayaka became the king in 1664. He was a young, handsome and virtuous prince and every noble in the court was busy searching for a suitable bride for him.

At the court in Bidanur, his elder ministers often argued, 'Maharaj, Keladi needs an heir. Is it not time for you to take a wife?' The powerful kingdoms of Swadi and Beelagi have offered the hands of their daughters. If you marry them, these alliances will make our kingdom stronger.'

The King listened to all of them patiently before rejecting their proposals. The people of Keladi, knowing his devotion to God, wondered whether their virtuous King would one day become a monk.

When the King went to the Rameshwara fair, his eyes fell on a very pretty girl buying dolls with her friends. For a few moments, the King's heart stopped beating; he was enchanted and he lost his peace of mind for the next few months.

For many days following that, the King remained pensive. His minister and close friend Veeranna decided to find out the reason.

'I cannot see you brooding all the day. What's the matter?' He asked Somashekhara.

'Veeranna, my friend, I am in love. You have been compelling me to marry for a long time. If I ever marry, I will marry only her.' The King narrated the incident to Veeranna.

Veeranna took charge of the situation and started searching for the girl. His search ended at the doors of Siddappa Shetty, a merchant of Kotepura.

'Maharaj, the Nayaka kings marry only among the royal bloods and she is only a commoner.'

'Veeranna, I shall either marry her or I won't marry at all.' The King was ready to abandon royal tradition for his love.

The humble merchant, the father of the girl, was amazed. He could not believe his fortune. Chennamma, his daughter, was obviously elated.

The wedding ceremony took place in the majestic palace of Bidanur with royal splendor.

Somashekhara loved Chennamma more than anything in the world. Perfectly complementing each other, the royal couple was a role model for the citizens. In a few months' time, Somashekhara transformed a doll-loving innocent but intelligent village girl into a regal lady with fine understanding of administration, and deftness in archery, horse riding and war-craft.

They were religious and joined their subjects in offering prayers at the temple of Lord Rameshwaram in Keladi, at Aghoreshwara temple in Ikkeri and at the Goddess Mookambike temple at Kollur. Both of them looked after the subjects together and ruled wisely.

The royal household was very happy but one thing was amiss; even after years of the marriage, the kingdom of Keladi was still waiting an heir.

Despite the murmuring in the palace and outside, and urgings to the King to remarry, Somashekhara never bothered. He was deeply in love with Chennamma.

At Bidanur, an influential noble, Bharama Mahuta was incharge of the royal elephants. Besides looking after the royal elephants, he also practised medicines, and was considered an expert in herbs and witchcraft. In fact, it was rumoured that he knew black magic and had employed many ghosts. Slowly, careful manipulation, he became an intimate friend to the king.

Since his youth, Mahuta had nurtured ambitions for Keladi's throne. Initially, he was very pleased with the King's decision to not marry, and seeing the happy couple later made him grudge their happiness and peace.

Executing a meticulous plan, Bharama Mahuta married a second time. His second wife was a beautiful woman with a grown-up daughter. His stepdaughter, Kalavathi, was a beautiful dancer and an excellent singer. When, in passing, during a momentary weakness, the King expressed his concerns over being childless, Bharama decided to take advantage of the king's weakness.

'Maharaj, the stress of public life is affecting your marital life. Your wise ancestors had therefore rightly encouraged the Dashahara tradition and started the Nadahabba cultural festival. You should watch this year's performances.'

The King agreed happily.

As per the plan, during that year's Nadahabba festival, Kalavathi presented her art before the King. Dancing like a peacock and singing like a cuckoo, she won the heart of Somashekhara. A highly pleased King not only showered gifts on her but also appointed her as the new royal court dancer.

Gradually, the frequency of Somashekhara's visit to Mahuta's residence increased under Bharama's encouragement. Kalavathi's beauty enchanted the King and he began to spend most of his time with her at Bharama's place, completely ignoring Chennamma and his duty as a king.

Bharama had hoped that Kalavathi would soon give the King his much-needed progeny but his hopes remained unfulfilled, and he decided to play a cruel trick to win the throne.

In the palace, the King's apathy had made Chennamma very sad; the King who once loved her so dearly, no more visited her. His indifference towards his duties had also begun to show. Unrest was brewing among the people who once sang paeans praising him. The kingdom was surely slipping into chaos and the disgruntled nobles started hatching conspiracies to usurp the throne.

Apart from these internal troubles, the threat from the Sultan of Bijapur was also looming large. Amidst this crisis, Veeranna decided to meet Chennamma.

'Devi, how can you be a mute spectator to this decay?' Veeranna challenged her. 'For more than 150 years, the Nayakas have ensured prosperity, peace and order in Keladi. In the past, we have defeated Bijapur many times and now it threatens to invade us? Nobles are raising their ignoble heads and the King has lost his way.' He looked into Chennamma's eyes and dared her, 'Devi, if you will remain passive, the legacy of the great Shivappa Nayaka will be lost.'

The Queen decided to put her pride aside and went to meet the King in the dancer's house. Kalavathi, Bharama Mahuta and a few of his friends were sitting around the King. Chennamma tried to convince the King in every possible way but deceived by the charm of Kalavathi, the guile of Bharama and the duplicity of his friends, the King refused to listen to Chennamma.

On her miserable return, the Queen called a meeting of few of her faithful nobles.

'For the dynasty to survive, we all have to run it together. On behalf of the King, I will supervise the day-to-day affairs of the state with your help,' she announced.

In those days of gloom, expecting such camaraderie was too much. The arrogant nobles thought that a woman could easily be frightened. Bharama thought it was the right time to play out his last act—further tempting the Sultan of Bijapur.

'Devi, it will be difficult for you to rule alone. I recommend you adopt Veerabhadra Nayaka, son of our army chief. We will all support you as a regent till he is able to run the kingdom,' Chief Minister Thimmanna Nayaka proposed.

'Devi, we don't agree with the Chief Minister,' many councillors shouted. 'But, we want young Shivappa Nayaka to be crowned as the king.'

'We don't agree with them,' a minister, Narsappayya, and an officer, Lakshamayya, argued. 'What is wrong with our children?'

Unperturbed by the chaos around her, the Queen closed the meeting, 'Nayakas, I will think over it and let you know.'

The nobles mistook the Queen's reply as her indecisiveness and began to plot against Chennamma herself.

'We will overthrow her. How can a merchant's daughter be our queen?'

'She does not have a single drop of royal blood in her veins. How could she preside over us?'

The nobles and the ministers decided to challenge the

Queen next day, in an open court.

There, in Kalavathi's house, sensing his slim chances of taking over the throne, Mahuta tried to convince the King.

'Maharaj, you need an heir to end this chaos. There is nothing in this world that cannot be cured. Our Vedas say that without fulfilling one's ancestor's debt, no one can proceed to heaven.'

'Yes, only the birth of a child ensures his parents a safe journey to heaven.'

'Lord, may I suggest a remedy?'

'Nothing can cure it,' the dejected King said.

Mahuta looked into the eyes of the King as if redemption was possible. The King lowered his eyes and meekly asked, 'What is this remedy you have?'

'Maharaj, it is made of the fluid that the elephant secretes during its mating season.'

The King looked at Bharama in disbelief.

'Don't worry.' Bharama Mahuta assured the King. 'It is an infallible remedy.' He paused and then added in a hushed tone, 'I agree that it is quite is unusual, so kindly speak of this to no one.'

The mating season was not very far.

Jannopant was a key advisor and confidant of the Sultan of Bijapur. Bharama Mahuta contacted him. The Sultan was already waiting for an opportunity to guzzle up the kingdom of Keladi. The prevailing situation at Keladi had presented too tempting an opportunity and he quickly sent Jannopant to the Queen for negotiations and also deployed his noble, Muzaffar Khan, to follow Jannopant with a huge army to annex Keladi, in case the negotiations fail.

Chennamma was perplexed; of late, she had put Bharama's house under surveillance and had come to know about Jannopant's secret meeting with Mahuta and of the Sultan's treacherous plot. One of her influential nobles, Kenga Hanumappa Nayak of Tarikere, also met Jannopant and offered his services. A helpless Queen was not in a position to counter these acts.

When Jannopant met her, a cornered Queen readily agreed to pay the sum demanded by the Sultan, and to all his other conditions. Despite these submissions, the Bijapur army's march had accelerated. The Queen was alerted and she tried to refuel her husband's sleepy conscience, while urging her people to support her against the enemy's onslaught.

That evening, she again visited the King.

'Maharaj, we are surrounded by the enemies.'

'But, I need an heir first, Chennamma. Even if I fight and win, the kingdom is useless without an heir.'

'What you say is true. But, all citizens are like children to a king. We have our responsibilities towards them as well. You should make them secure and happy. You are the father...'

'Father?' A violent Somashekhara snapped at her, 'Why do you mock me with that word, Chennamma?'

With that, the King got up and went straight into Kalavathi's bedroom.

'If you do not execute your duties, I will do mine towards my people,' a teary-eyed Chennamma shouted at his back.

When Jannopant and Bharama heard about the Queen's resolve to fight the Sultan's army, they decided to bring down the curtains faster.

'Bharama, is it ready?' The King had no other thoughts

in his mind.

'Lord, yes. The elephant remedy is ready,' Mahuta offered him the blend.

The solution had a quick reaction and with a loud cry Somashekhara fell on the ground and died.

The Queen knew who was behind the king's murder.

Chennamma raided Mahuta's house with her trusted soldiers and got him arrested.

'Bury this snake in a pit,' she ordered. 'Take him to an isolated place and burn him the way he burnt down my happy home.'

She returned to the royal court and assembled all the people of Keladi.

'People of Keladi, you have heard the news. Keladi is under attack. Our first job is to repel the invader.'

'But first, we should decide who will lead us. Who will be the new king?' Chief Minister Thimmanna Nayaka demanded.

'Right now, it is not important. We have to counter the Sultan's army first.'

Hearing the Queen's reply, the Chief Minister began to walk out.

'Thimmanna, wait. Keladi needs you in her hour of crisis.'

'I cannot stay in a kingdom that does not have a ruler,' Thimmanna walked out of the court.

Without batting an eyelid, the Queen addressed her people and soldiers.

'Brave men of Keladi, our beloved motherland, nurtured and handed down to us by our ancestors, is in danger. Is not it our duty to safeguard it?'

'Yes, it is,' everyone shouted back in response.

'Don't think of me as a queen,' Chennamma raised her pitch. 'Think of me as the voice of the great Shivappa Nayaka and the voice of my late husband, Somashekhara. It is their spirit which asks you to fight for the motherland.'

With this, she shed all her jewels and distributed them among her soldiers. She opened the treasury and distributed its wealth among her citizens.

'All this is payment for your war efforts,' she raised a sword high in the air, 'And these hands will now take up the sword to fight along with you.'

The Queen's words electrified the assembly. Everyone shouted her in support, 'We will fight. We will fight.'

An elated and spirited army of Keladi marched against the much larger army of Bijapur.

In the state capital of Bidanur, her faithful nobles counselled Chennamma.

'Your Highness, even if we fight with valour, our victory is doubtful. Let us vacate Bidanur for the time being.'

'No. That will be cowardice.'

For her, the mere thought of leaving Bidanur was terrible.

'Don't you remember Ranchhod Krishna?' Veeranna asked, 'It's a temporary move. Let the throne, royal treasury and other valuables be moved to Bhuvanagiri. The fortress there is situated amidst thick jungles and is secure.'

There, in the battleground, the small Keladi army could resist Bijapur, but briefly. The Sultan's army soon entered the town and captured the fort. When Muzaffar Khan entered the palace, he found it empty.

'An empty city! Where is everyone?' He shouted at his deputy.

After a little search, they only found an elderly caretaker; there was no doubt that the town had been evacuated purposefully.

'Where is the throne? Where is your woman-ruler? Where are the jewels?' An angry Muzaffar Khan shouted and pressed his knife against the old man's throat. 'Where is the treasury?'

'Gone. You can never find them,' the old caretaker laughed and exposed his bare chest.

Meanwhile, Chennamma had taken refuge in Bhuvanagiri.

'We did right,' she told herself, 'It would have been foolish to sacrifice everything. We should begin preparations to recapture the lost capital.'

One evening, Veeranna knocked at her door. She opened it apprehensively, expecting to hear some bad news. He was standing with Thimmanna Nayaka, the chief minister who had abandoned the Queen on the issue of succession.

'You?' The Queen was surprised.

'Mahadevi,' Thimmanna apologized, 'I am guilty of an unpardonable crime. I deserted Keladi, when it needed me most.' The old warrior wiped his tears. 'I feel ashamed to even ask for your forgiveness. Bidanur's fall into foreign hands have broken my heart. Please accept me back into your services.'

'Thimmanna, how can we believe you?' Veeranna taunted.

'Wait Veeranna…' Chennamma proudly looked at the warrior.

'Thimmanna, the sun of Keladi's fortune has not set yet. How can we forget the services rendered by you in the past.'

Without wasting time, Chennamma appointed him her commander-in-chief. Thimmanna worked with a greater zeal and organized the soldiers and citizens, and trained them hard.

The news of Thimmanna's coming back and training of volunteers spread like wild fire and people from all corners of the kingdom flocked in to Bhuvanagiri. The highly spirited people were ready to sacrifice their all for the kingdom and the Queen. Thimmanna was training the villagers and turning them into a band of courageous soldiers.

An alerted Bijapur army located the Queen's hideout and marched towards Bhuvanagiri.

The Queen was more than ready for it.

'Soldiers, the enemy is marching towards us. You know this terrain like the back of your palm. Use the terrain, hit the enemy and run away. Keep repeating it till we finish them off.'

Amidst thick forests and narrow passes, the heroic Keladi warriors destroyed the sultan's soldiers. Proceeding to Bidanur, the Queen, with her victorious soldiers, freed their capital. Jannopant was captured and put to death.

In 1671, amidst the cheering and an over joyous crowd, Chennamma was crowned the queen of Keladi.

Keladi's administration had suffered a lot in past few years. Chaos and misrule had emptied the treasury. Chennamma took over the entire administration in her hands. She reinforced the administrative system formulated by Shivappa Nayaka and expanded her army and strengthened the security of the borders. She encouraged sea trade by utilizing Keladi's long seacoast and established profitable trade routes with the Arabs, the Portuguese, the Dutch and the English for valuable Arab horses and military ammunition, in exchange of high quality pepper and rice that grew in Keladi. By her hard work and welfare measures, she brought peace and happiness back in Keladi.

After bringing peace in Ikkeri, Chennamma subdued Ramchandra Nayaka of Sode, Karakala and Mallikarjuna, and also Kasaragod. Jealous neighbours and disgruntled local chieftains began to hatch conspiracies against the prosperous Keladi and its popular queen.

Chikkadevaraya Wodeyar, the king of Mysore, attacked Keladi. Rebelling Keladi chieftains like Andhaka Venkata Nayaka, lords of large villages like Sode, Sirsi and Banvasi, and many other neighbouring kings joined Mysore's ranks to oust the woman ruler.

Chikkadevaraya thought it to be quite easy to defeat an army led by a woman; he was highly mistaken. Chennamma remained undaunted and sent a huge army under her commander, Bhadrappa Nayaka to fight the enemy. A fierce war followed and in the end, the Queen very cleverly managed to defeat her enemies.

It was a humiliating defeat for Wodeyar. Next year, he again attacked Keladi and but this time he emerged victorious. But, in the third war, Chennamma defeated him again and captured many top officers of the Mysore army. At the end of the war, she released all war prisoners and sent them back to Mysore. Everyone praised her humanitarian treatment of the war prisoners and Chikkadevaraya offered her a treaty of friendship.

After her victory over Mysore, Chennmma also defeated a combined force of rebellious chieftains of Keladi.

After narrating the story of Chennamma of Keladi, Tara Bai looked at Rajaram.

'So, she does not have an heir to the throne?' Rajaram asked.

'Chennamma has adopted a child, Basava. She is grooming him to be her successor.' Tara Bai paused and then said, 'Chhatrapati, you can trust her.'

A convinced Rajaram fled before the Mughals could capture him.

Meanwhile, in Keladi, almost two decades of Chennamma's rule had brought lasting peace. She had begun a tradition of giving alms to the needy every afternoon and followed that religiously.

One day, during her daily alms giving session, she noticed four monks waiting in a corner. The monks waited till everyone else received their alms and left. The Queen realized that the monks were not ordinary beggars.

When the Queen gave alms to the chief monk, he blessed her.

'You are no ordinary man,' the Queen said, 'Why have you embraced a monk's life at such a young age?'

'I am no monk, mother,' Rajaram looked at her face and then at her feet, 'I am like your son.'

'True. My child, tell me what can I do for you?'

'I am Rajaram, son of Chhatrapati Shivaji,' he revealed his identity. 'Aurangzeb's army is chasing me. I want to go to Jinji to consolidate my position. But no king is ready to help me fearing Aurangzeb. I need your shelter for a few days and then your help in reaching Jinji.'

She kept on looking at him affectionately. A baffled

Rajaram enquired, 'Mother, if you fear the wrath of Aurangzeb, I won't bother you.'

'Son, you mock me in putting so much effort in your request. I am a mother and the queen of Keladi. It is my duty to protect you.'

But, it was not so easy. Most of her chiefs, including Veeranna and Thimmanna opposed her.

'Mahadevi, please forgive me. But, we will never be able to stand up to the might of the Mughals,' Thimmanna opined.

'If Aurangzeb comes to know, he will ensure our complete ruin,' Veeranna supported his colleague.

Even, the Queen's father, Siddappa Shetty, cautioned her, 'After many years of turbulence, peace and order have returned to Keladi. Don't upset it.'

Almost all the courtiers were of the same opinion.

'What do you say, Basava?' The Queen turned to her young son.

'Mother, your decision to give protection to Chhatrapati is correct and in line with Keladi's glorious tradition,' Basava supported her.

'Thimanna, let us prepare for the war,' the Queen decided.

When Aurangzeb came to know about Rajaram's presence in Keladi, he sent a huge army under Jaan Nisar Khan to march to Keladi. Simultaneously, the Emperor sent a messenger to the royal court of Keladi. But before the messenger could reach Bidanur, Rajaram had safely reached Jinji.

'Alamgir Aurangzeb, the greatest emperor, greets you, Your Highness. He demands that you should give away his enemy Rajaram to him without delay. Only then, you will avoid the destruction that a hostile Mughal army can unleash.'

The Queen smiled and drafted a reply.

'Emperor, Rajaram is no longer in Keladi. It is of course known that he passed through Keladi in the garb of a monk.'

By the time her reply reached the Emperor, the Mughal army had already attacked Keladi and entered the kingdom.

The Queen was well prepared for the war. The path to Bidanur lay through a thick jungle and the monsoons had set in. Once the Mughals were within the thick webs of the Malenadu forests, Chennamma's soldiers put into use their old tactic of using the terrain, hitting the enemy and running away. They broke Mughal confidence and harassed them to no end. For them, passing through the thick maze of jungles in a heavy downpour became extremely difficult. Keladi's warriors had taken positions in the familiar jungles and butchered the Mughal army. They captured many Mughal officers and seized a large number of their horses and ammunition.

In that embarrassing moment when an epidemic and leeches were killing as many soldiers as the Keladi warriors had killed, Jaan Nisar Khan got a relieving message from Aurangzeb.

'There is no fun in wasting time in Malenadu jungles. Rajaram has reached Jinji. Change your course and move straight to Jinji.'

The Mughals called for peace. Chennamma quickly accepted it. Rajaram had been saved by then.

Chennamma ruled for twenty-five years. Her reign is remembered for her efficient rule, justice, and generosity. She built many schools, ponds and temples. Basava Nayaka, her adopted son, had come of age. Before her death, she took a promise from her son.

'Basava, we could not have wished for a finer son than you. Son, always keep your word and never neglect your duty. Do not tread an unworthy path and don't differentiate between your kinsfolk. Son, two more things, live as an object of people's praise and strive to know yourself.'

Master in statecraft, Basava Nayaka proved to be an able successor to Chennamma. In her heydays, Chennamma had won a ruined fort at Hulikere near Basavapuram and got it rebuilt. When Basava became the king, he renamed it 'Chennagiri' in honour of his mother. He also wrote the fine Kannada text *Shivatatva Ratnakara* and dedicated it to his mother.

Tara Bai

'Bhadrakali had lost.' She pitied herself in that darkest hour of Maratha history. Staring at the vacuum outside her Satara palace balcony, eighty-six years old Tara Bai saw Chhatrapati Shivaji's dream disappearing without a trace.

'Me, Bhadrakali?' The dowager queen of the Marathas, Tara Bai Bhonsle, spat out in frustration. News of the massacre of more than one lakh Marathas reached Satara before the northern winds, and told the ignoble story of what happened on 14 January 1761 at Panipat.

A stunned Tara Bai looked at the tired messenger. 'How could it be possible?' The entire generation of legendary Maratha warriors and the generation after had been wiped away by Ahmad Shah Abdali's Afghan forces.

Tara Bai's thoughts went back to the day when the Marathas had taken control of the Mughal capital Dilli on 2 August 1760, after leaving Patdurg on 14 March 1760 at a leisurely pace.

Leisurely pace! Yes, the slow-moving Maratha camp took four and a half months to reach Dilli. 'Unthinkable for any army moving to capture Hindustan!' In contrast, the Marathas under her were often compared to hyenas closing in on the dying lion, when they hounded Aurangzeb.

In 1760, the Maratha power was at its zenith, but the character of its campaigns had changed. The over confident and arrogant Maratha army had moved with 300,000 non-combatants including servants, maids, entertainers, pilgrims, tourists, children and camp followers. Little skirmishes with Afghans became the norm once the Marathas occupied Dilli. A battle between the two forces took place at Kunjpura. The Marathas defeated 15,000 strong Afghans. This small victory made the Marathas complacent and they began to treat Dilli and Panipat as Pune.

'They ignored my warnings.' She rued. 'I advised Sadashivrao Bhau to not take the entire city with him. But, just like the other peshwas, he did not listen to me.' She looked at the messenger urging for more details.

'During the festive season, Abdali daringly crossed River Yamuna at Baghpat, cutting off the Maratha camp from its base in Dilli. This move fell heavy on the Marathas in the town of Panipat. The siege ran for two months while both the sides tried cutting off each other's supplies. Abdali, however, outsmarted the Marathas in that game and by the end of November 1760, he cut off all the food supplies into the besieged camp, which had about 300,000 non-combatants. By late December, food in the Maratha camp ran out and the cattle died by the thousands. The Gregorian new year saw the soldiers dying of starvation. On 13 January 1761, the Maratha commanders begged Commander Bhau to allow them to die on the battleground than to perish by starvation.

'Next day, the Marathas attacked the Afghan camp in a desperate attempt to break the siege. War began in the morning and continued till the evening. Around 70,000 soldiers died in the battle and 40,000 Maratha prisoners were slaughtered in cold blood.'

Till her death, later that year, Tara Bai could not reconcile with the news. 'Never was a defeat so complete and never would there be a calamity which diffused so much consternation.'

The grand dream of Shivaji had shattered and before they could realize it, the Marathas had vacated the throne of India for a new power, the British.

When against all odds, Shivaji was formally crowned as Chhatrapati, the king, at Raigarh in 1674 during the heydays of the Mughal Emperor Aurangzeb, the nascent state was destined to be always at odds with the Mughals.

During these battles with the Mughals, a crafty and gallant commander Hambirrao Mohite ably supported Shivaji. He later became the commander-in-chief of the Maratha army and his daughter, Tara Bai, was given in marriage to Shivaji's second son, Rajaram, at a very young age. Rajaram's mother Soyra Bai was Shivaji's second wife and also an aunt of Tara Bai.

The question of succession became complicated even during Shivaji's lifetime. His eldest son and heir-apparent Shambhuji was an irresponsible man and addicted to sensual pleasures. When Shivaji confined him to curb his ill habits, Shambhuji defected to the Mughals. After enjoying Mughal hospitality for one year, he returned without a trace of repentance.

Shivaji's death from fever and dysentery, at an age of 52, was followed by a lot of rumours. Within a month of Shivaji's death, Soyra Bai installed her ten-year-old son Rajaram on the throne.

However, with the help of a faction of the ministers, Shambhuji acquired control of Raigarh and imprisoned Rajaram and Soyra Bai. After a few months, he executed Soyra Bai on charges of conspiracy.

During these troubled times, Tara Bai's father, Hambirrao Mohite managed to stabilize the Maratha ship by siding with Shambhuji, instead of Rajaram.

'Tara, I was born in a poor farmer family at Talbid near Satara. I have followed Shivaji Maharaj through thick and thin. He taught me that posts, perks and privileges are temporary things. Who becomes the king or queen is not important. The only thing that matters is replacing the Mughals as the rulers of Hindustan.'

Mohite looked affectionately at his very young daughter, the wife of the ten-year-old dethroned king Rajaram, and then said, 'Tara, I trust Shambhuji to lead the Marathas ahead.'

The following years saw the Maratha army invading one kingdom after another. The winning caravan's last trophy was Burhanpur which was plundered by Shambhuji and his men.

'Chhatrapati, this goes against Shivaji Maharaj's policies. We never do this. The late Maharaj had prohibited torture and violence on defeated enemy and the residents,' Mohite protested.

Shambhuji laughed cruelly. 'Mohite, if you saw the Mughal torture, you would have not said that.'

This was the beginning of Shambhuji's decline.

Under Shambhuji, the Marathas waged many unsuccessful campaigns against the Mughals. They could also not succeed against the Siddies of Janjira and the king of Mysore.

With every unsuccessful campaign, Mohite became more frustrated. He realized that Shambhuji was not a visionary like Shivaji. He was cruel and his sensual fancies had grown increasingly dangerous in the company of the royal poet, Kavi Kalash.

That was in 1687, and Tara Bai had started understanding the Maratha politics. She was a spirited girl and had an intelligent mind.

'Are we going to war without preparation?' she asked her father.

'No, we are taking about 50,000 men. But, the Mughals may bring around one million.'

'One million?' she gasped.

Her father smiled, 'Tara, Aurangzeb is the most powerful emperor in the world. They call him *aalamgir*. He has been in Deccan since the last decade only to crush the Marathas. He decimated the strong Bijapur and Golkunda empires in no time.'

'I fear Shirke...' she whispered.

'The Shirkes are not to be trusted. I told the Chhatrapati, but he hardly pays heed to my caution.'

Both father and daughter remained silent for a long time. Then Mohite stated a fact: 'The Jadhavas and the Shirkes may fight on the Mughal side against us.'

A few weeks later, the Maratha and the Mughal armies met at Wai, near Satara. A cannonball struck Mohite during the war and seeing him fall, the Maratha army lost its morale.

The Battle of Wai weakened the Maratha power immensely; the troops started deserting Shambhuji. The Shirkes were spying on him and reported his every movement to Aurangzeb.

In February 1689, Shambhuji was captured at Sangameshwar.

At Bahadurgarh, Aurangzeb paraded Shambhuji and Kavi Kalash in clown's clothes and subjected them to insults by the Mughal soldiers. When Shambhuji refused to convert to Islam, Aurangzeb ordered both of them to be tortured to death. The torture continued for a fortnight which included plucking out their eyes and tongues, pulling out their nails and removing their skin. The Mughals did not stop here. Shambhuji's body was torn apart with *wagh nakh*—metal tiger claws—and finally he was beheaded with an axe at Talpur near Pune.

Shambhuji's brutal end put the Maratha confederacy into disarray. Tara Bai acted swiftly and convinced an indecisive Rajaram to assume the throne.

'We will maintain our dignity and freedom. The Mughals are inching closer to Raigarh. Jinji remains our only hope. The Chhatrapati Rajaram should go there and consolidate the Maratha position,' she advised her husband.

'How can I reach Jinji? No king will help me and make enemies out of the Mughals,' a shaken Rajaram said.

'Queen Chennamma of Keladi can help you reach Jinji,' Tara Bai was very sure and convinced Rajaram.

Rajaram escaped in time. Within a few days, Raigarh fell into the hands of the Mughals and Yesubai and Shambhuji's son, Shahu, were captured.

With the help of Santaji Ghorpade, Tara Bai escaped to the nearby hills, where she reorganized the Maratha guerilla fighters.

'I vow, I will not allow peace to the Mughals.'

'Aai, we are with you,' said Santaji Ghorpade and Dhanaji Jadhav, two bitter rivals yet legendary Maratha generals, declared their loyalty to Tara Bai.

'Meticulous planning, rapid movement, precise timing and coordination will be the key. Let our planning and executions be such that no Mughal amir is bold enough to resist them, and every move of ours should make the bravest enemy warrior quake.'

'It will be so,' Santaji and Dhanaji vowed.

Together, they assembled few hundred soldiers and launched guerilla attacks on the Mughals.

A charged Santaji managed to negotiate the River Bhima despite floods and attacked the Mughal camp at Tulapur with 2,000 soldiers. Though the Marathas were in small numbers, their attack was fierce and focused.

In a daring feat, Santaji cut the ropes of Aurangzeb's tents and took the imperial golden pinnacle and fled. They killed many of Aurangzeb's commanders, though the Mughal Emperor survived. The Marathas had become the terror for the Mughals. Everyone who encountered them was either killed or wounded or imprisoned; the enemy barely managed to escape alive.

Aurangzeb was furious. 'Few mountain rats are daring to trouble us. I am ashamed of my generals.'

His deputy Ghazi-ud-din Firoze Jung tried to bring down the spirit of the Tara Bai by numerous attempts to capture her. But the alert Queen escaped his clutches every time.

The Mughals had chased Rajaram right from Raigarh. Few months after Rajaram's arrival, Zulfiqar Khan, a general of Aurangzeb, sieged the fort of Jinji. Tara Bai was not getting any help from Rajaram, who had virtually become a prisoner in Jinji.

A worried Tara Bai sent a message to her husband.

'Zulfiqar has the power to destroy all the Marathas in the country. He is very ambitious. He does not like idly sitting in the royal court, but enjoys battle camps where he wields enormous power. Try to mould him to go for tangential campaigns.'

If Zulfiqar had wished, he could have captured Jinji in one day, but he wanted to prolong the operation. Thus, encouraged by Rajaram, he decided to plan for his own principality in the Deccan, counting on the imminent death of an old Aurangzeb.

This went on for seven years. Finally, a frustrated Aurangzeb pressed hard on his general to produce results. Zulfiqar stormed Jinji, but not before warning Rajaram about his intended action so that the Chhatrapati could escape.

Tara Bai found Rajaram subdued on his return. He was tired of the constant Mughal chasing and siege. With his increasing depression, he soon fell ill. His health began deteriorating gradually as he began to spit blood and suffered from inflammation of the lungs.

The Marathas were under severe crisis again. Shambhuji's son Shahu was the Mughal prisoner and Rajaram's son Shivaji II was a newborn.

On 3 March 1700, Rajaram died. Many Maratha chiefs, including Dhanaji Jadhav, abhorred the idea of a lady regent. They placed Rajaram's illegitimate son Raja Karna on the throne, thus, dividing the Marathas again. However, Raja Karna died of small pox within three weeks. Without wasting time on tears, Tara Bai proclaimed her four-year-old son Shivaji

II as the new Maratha king and took the reins of the kingdom in her hands. Though it looked like the star of the Maratha power was on a decline after the fall of Satara, its capital city, in April 1700, Tara Bai took rigorous measures to ravage the Mughal territory.

'There seems to be no end to this dark tunnel. But, pradhans, I assure you, one day we will find the light and the Marathas will rule over Hindustan.' Tara Bai addressed the Maratha pradhans.

No one shared her belief and conviction.

'Aurangzeb calls us hill rats. Let us make holes in the Mughal confidence. I will ensure that Aurangzeb's grave gets dug in Deccan. We will plot his and the Mughal empire's downfall. We cannot fight them in a direct battle. We will surprise them with our small but intense attacks from all directions. They will not know when, how and where we will attack. Let us spread like ants and locusts throughout the Deccan.'

'How?' her minister Parasuram Trimbak asked.

'The way our commanders did. Let us ride on the wave of this Maratha insurgency. Let us penetrate into the Mughal territories, wherever they want. Let them plunder and destroy the Mughal dominions.'

'It will create chaos,' someone protested.

'Initially, yes. Slowly, out of this chaos will emerge a military confederacy, which I will link to the central authority.'

'How?'

'The servants of the Maratha state will support themselves by plundering on all sides, and pay *chauth* to their king, getting no salary from them. I will distribute the whole empire among my generals.'

Very soon, Tara Bai launched a series of Parthian style attacks on the Mughals. She exhibited wonderful powers of organization and planning. Aurangzeb directed his forces to win Panhala and Vishalgarh, the two seats of the Maratha court. Tara Bai quickly moved back but constantly hovered around the Emperor's camp and the Marathas carried away everything that they could. Aurangzeb captured several Maratha forts, but only to lose them one by one.

Despite all his campaigns and the endless sieges, Aurangzeb failed to stop the Maratha juggernaut. Under the leadership of Tara Bai, the Marathas were growing stronger and Aurangzeb was compelled to be on the defensive. Within three years, he understood that he was losing the big game in Deccan. He opened talks with Dhanaji to handover Shahu to him.

'This is a ploy to divide us,' Tara Bai was furious.

'I know,' Dhanaji replied. 'I will put forth extravagant demands.'

Tara Bai looked at her army chief with suspicion but said nothing. She had the larger cause in her heart.

Aurangzeb did not agree to the Maratha demands. However, the negotiations themselves proved to be a big morale-boosting win for the Marathas.

In 1705, Tara Bai sent a Maratha army of 40,000 soldiers to Gujarat, following which a huge area of Gujarat up to Bharuch came under the Maratha dominion. Very soon, the Nawab of Vadodara, Nazar Ali was defeated and the Maratha empire extended till Vadodara.

The following year, Tara Bai extended her territories up to southern Mysore. She proceeded beyond Maharashtra and led distant expeditions across the River Narmada into Malwa and Gujarat. The Marathas emerged victorious after a drawn-out and fiercely fought battle, effectively ending the Mughal dominance in Deccan.

The Marathas raided the Mughal territory up to Ahmedabad. This caused serious territorial as well as prestigious damage to the Mughals and its aged Emperor. Her triumphs forced the Mughal historian Khafi Khan to write, 'She was the only lady capable of taking over six provinces of the Mughal Empire, a great feat indeed.'

Tara Bai made life frustratingly hard for the Mughals during the last six years of Aurangzeb's life. Such was the Mughal grind in living in tents for decades that a homesick general even offered to pay Aurangzeb 100,000 rupees for permission to spend a year in Dilli.

For a man rarely accustomed to failure, Aurangzeb had to bear the ignominy of repeated failures. The Maratha rats were raiding everywhere and amidst their persistent attacks, Aurangzeb breathed his last as a bitter man, at Aurangabad, in 1707.

The Mughals could not bear this loss and released Prince Shahu from their captivity to create dissension in the Maratha ranks. Tara Bai understood the politics very well and refused to acknowledge Shahu as the real king. But, many Maratha generals joined hands with Shahu.

'You should also join Shahuji Maharaj,' Dhanaji's young assistant, Balaji Vishwanath advised him. 'Shahu is the son of Shambhuji and therefore our natural leader. Tara Bai is just a custodian.'

Nodding his head in agreement, Dhanaji thought hard and then asked his young assistant to mediate.

Defection of her army chief weakened the position of Tara Bai considerably. Except Parasuram Trimbak, all her lieutenants had deserted her.

But, she was not someone to go down easily. She waged many conflicts against Shahu but desertion of her closest aides was weakening her day by day. Finally, after the defeat at Khed, she reluctantly agreed to accept Shahu as the rightful king of the Marathas.

'I still hold my head high, son.' She said, 'May you complete the unfinished task of Shivaji Maharaj and unfurl the Hindu Pad Padshahi pataka at the Red Fort.'

'I will work for that, Aai. Without your exertions the fledgling Maratha kingdom would not have survived the reign of Aurangzeb,' a magnanimous Shahu allowed her to retire to the province of Kolhapur.

Tara Bai established an independent throne at Kolhapur in 1713. Despite being humbled by Shahu, her ambitions were yet to be subdued. She continued her scheming against Shahu.

A daughter of hereditary landlords and military men, the Deshmukhs, Tara Bai was now pitted against a sharp Brahmin peshwa, Balaji Vishwanath, whose ancestors were rooted in the finance and banking.

Balaji Vishwanath, now the peshwa of Shahu, successfully halted her plans. He helped Rajaram's other wife, Rajasbai, and her son Shambhuji II to usurp the throne of Kolhapur. Rajasbai imprisoned Tara Bai. But, Shambhuji II proved a weak king. He began conspiracies along with Nizam Chin Quli Khan against Shahu. As a result, Shahu's armies defeated and forced him to give up all the territories north of the River Warna. Shahu also released Tara Bai and allowed her to stay in the palace of Satara.

By then, the institution of the peshwas had become very strong and hereditary. None other than the strongest peshwa ever, Balaji Bajirao was running the Maratha confederacy. Tara Bai had always felt that the peshwas had appropriated powers that her own father-in-law Shivaji, had invested only in the Maratha Chhatrapati.

Tara Bai tried to remove Bajirao from his post, but failed. Ironically, as much as Tara Bai resented and plotted against the peshwas, the peshwas became more powerful and supreme. In 1749, before his death, Shahu voluntarily delegated considerable power to the Peshwa.

After the death of an heirless Shahu, Tara Bai presented Rajaram II as a more direct descendent and who had a greater right to succeed Shahu. She introduced him as her grandson whom everyone had thought had died. Tara Bai reasoned that she had kept him hidden to save him from assassination attempts.

Now through Rajaram II, Tara Bai tried to exercise control over the affairs of the Maratha kingdom. But, very soon irreconcilable disputes created enmity between the two. As a result, Tara Bai imprisoned Rajaram II rendering him ineffectual and also denied that he was her grandson. Thus, she deprived him of a legitimate claim to the throne. This naturally enhanced the authority of the peshwa and undermined the chhatrapati's.

After a brief power struggle between Peshwa Balaji Bajirao and Tara Bai, eventually power shifted decisively to the Peshwa.

Now, the much old Tara Bai agreed and accepted the ultimate power of the peshwas and in return got the independent control over her principality, Kolhapur. Rajaram remained her prisoner till the end.

Darkness had descended. The old Queen knew that even the era of the peshwas was about to end.

'Not only the peshwas but the dream of a Maratha Hindustan is over. Europeans are the new kingmakers.' She sighed.

She remembered *Ajnapatra*.

Long ago, in 1715, she had asked her chief advisor, Ramchandra Nilkanth, to complete a political treatise. He named it *Ajnapatra* and discussed various topics in it, including the arrival of Europeans in the western Deccan.

'They wear a strange hat, Aai,' Nilkanth said.

'They are harmless ordinary merchants,' she remarked.

'I beg your pardon, Aai,' Nilkanth protested, 'they may appear to be ordinary merchants, but they are not. Their masters, every one of them, are reigning kings...'

'What are you saying?' she queried.

'These hat-wearers have ambitions to enter our provinces to increase their territories and to establish their own religion.' Nilkanth had said.

Now, the dying Queen understood what Nilkanth had said. 'In the last five decades, the "hat-wearers" have been swarming along the Indian shores like locusts. Some had already begun nibbling at the Indian territories, typically by marketing their weapons to the political players in the interior.'

She remembered an incident of April 1758 that should have opened her eyes.

In April 1758, the acting governor of Portuguese Goa had written to her that he would be pleased to supply her with the 2,000 guns she had ordered, provided she paid for them before the delivery.

The eighty-six years old dowager Queen closed her eyes not to ever open them again; the era of the 'hat-wearers' had dawned.

Chennamma of Kittur

'Baba, why do you address the Peshwa as Maharaj? Is he a king?' nine-year-old Manu asked her father, Moropant.

They were returning from Peshwa Bajirao II's mansion at Bithur, near Kanpur. Manu was a friend of the Peshwa's adopted son, Dhundhu, and Moropant was in service of the exiled Peshwa.

'Manu, when he became the peshwa in 1796, he was the maharaj of the Marathas.'

'Then what happened?'

'Then came the British,' Moropant took a long pause as if trying to gather his thoughts.

'Manu, only thirty-five years before Baji Rao's accession, the peshwas were the ruler of Hindustan. Unfortunately, two consequent events changed the course of the Maratha history.

After the death of the Peshwa Madhava Rao in 1772, a complex succession crisis started that ended the Maratha hegemony. Secondly, at around the same time, the British defeated a weak Mughal emperor at Baksar. The defeat was so decisive that it put an end to the Mughal history. The Marathas had even wanted to keep a token Mughal ruler in Delhi, as the former did not have a nation-wide presence, but this defeat aborted all Maratha attempts to revive it. A new race of conquerors began their career in India.'

The natural Maratha pride boiled inside the little girl. 'Baba, why could the great Maratha warriors not defeat a handful of foreigners?'

'They were businessmen and we were just haughty sword wagers,' Moropant remarked.

A puzzled Manu looked at her father.

'The British first made us believe that they were our friends in our battles against our own countrymen. When we began to lose our strength, they changed sides and attacked us. The succession crisis of the peshwa helped them; they supported any faction that would agree to their demands. By 1800, the last of the great Maratha leaders including Mahadji Scindia, Nana Phadnavis and Ahalyabai Holkar had died, bringing an end to the wisdom and moderation typical of the Maratha rulers. A fight for the control of the new Peshwa broke out between Yashwant Rao Holkar and Daulat Rao Scindia; this scared the present Peshwa Baji Rao and he fled across the Ghats, down to the coast and then into the open arms of the British.'

'Baba, are the British unconquerable?'

Moropant looked at her little daughter and remembered two great women rulers, Rani Ahalyabai Holkar and the Queen Chennamma of Kittur, who had, in the past, pondered upon the same question.

'Manu, the British are different. To win, they will not ravage your countryside and plunder your cities. They are so restrained in their language and so disciplined on field that they can even make hostility look like friendship and conquest like a favour.'

'Then how can they be defeated?'

'Only when you wage a direct and ruthless war against them, with firepower equal to or more than them.'

'I will do that.'

Moropant laughed at her childish vow.

'Manu, a queen tried that a few decades ago. But failed.'

'Tell me about her, Baba.'

Kittur or Kitturu is a small village in Mysore. It's near two important towns, Belgaum and Bailhongal. The Kittur kingdom was founded in 1585 by a Maratha Desai.

Mallasarja was the eleventh Desai of Kittur and was an ambitious ruler and a great warrior. In those days, for small principalities like Kittur, the fight for survival was intense. Three big powers ruled the Deccan and the south—the Marathas under the Peshwa, the Nizam of Hyderabad, and Haider Ali and his son, Tipu of Mysore. They were always looking for opportunities to usurp Kittur.

After Haider Ali's death, his son, Tipu was enthroned in 1783. Though the East India Company was constantly hounding him, Tipu kept on resisting their advances.

In 1788, he waged a fierce war with Kittur. At that time, Tipu was at the prime of his power and his ammunition factories at Bednur were producing 20,000 muskets and guns every year.

In that war of unequal powers, Mysore defeated Kittur and Mallasarja was captured and imprisoned. Tipu chained his prized prisoner in a cell on the top floor of his fort at Srirangapattanam. Mallasarja however had no intentions of being in chains for too long. With deft manipulation he influenced the royal guards to open his chains. Once freed, he managed to break the cell and scale down the elevated walls of the fort.

When the entire army of Tipu was searching for Mallasarja, he was living in a local temple in Srirangapattanam, dressed like a mendicant. His escape from Mysore became a legend story in Kittur.

Mallasarja was married to Rudramma, a kind-hearted queen and a simple soul. Their married life was a happy one. After his escape from Tipu's prison, once when he was touring the countryside, he met Chennamma for the first time.

She was only fifteen years old then and Mallasarja was the father of a ten-year-old prince, Shivalinga Rudrasarja.

Chennamma, like other girls of her age, had grown up hearing Mallasarja's tales of bravery. Her father, Dhoolappa Gowda, was an affluent Desai of Kagati. She had spent her childhood in the small fort of Kagati, where her parents not only instilled a lot of value but also trained her in horse riding, archery and sword fighting. Tales of her bravery were well known and they reached Mallasarja.

Mallasarja relentlessly pursued her father to convince him in giving his daughter in marriage to him. The marriage ceremony took place in the fort of Kagati with a lot of pomp and splendour. Mallasarja then returned to Kittur with his young bride.

'Chennamma, now onwards only Kittur will be your home and the king your only guardian. Serve both of them with whole hearted devotion,' a tearful Dhoolappa Gowda gave his daughter a final advice.

Contrary to Chennamma's expectations, when the newlyweds reached Kittur, Rudramma welcomed them with a lot of warmth and affection. Very soon, the queens became friends and even Shivalinga liked the beautiful, soft-spoken and loving Chennamma, who gladly took the responsibility of bringing him up. Chennamma introduced him to the scriptures and mathematics, and trained him in archery and sword fighting. The Mallasarja household was very happy to have Chennamma.

'He is learning what I wasn't able to teach him,' Rudramma affectionately praised Chennamma. 'Seeing you two, no one will believe that you are not his real mother.'

'Akka, I am also his mother. I wish and pray that he earns a name even bigger than his father,' Chennamma politely replied.

After a few years, Chennamma also gave birth to a son. The birth was celebrated with great fanfare, and every family in Kittur was invited to the boy's naming ceremony. Rudramma affectionately named him Basavaraja, or the Lord of Bulls, one of the many names of Lord Shiva.

Despite the difference in their ages, the princes forged an intimate bond. Through the years, the people of Kittur admired the young queen, who was equally at ease in the royal court as well as amongst peasants. In times of drought, Chennamma used to supervise the supply of grains from the royal granary to the homes of the needy. She also helped in the rehabilitation of the African slaves brought to India by the Portuguese. The Queen allowed them freedom in their lifestyles and provided new employment. She was respectful and tolerant towards everyone and was known to have renovated many dilapidated mosques in and around Kittur.

As a result, the people affectionately called her 'mother'.

Mallasarja now started arranging the weddings of the two princes—the elder prince Shivalinga Rudrasarja was married to Veeramma and Basavaraja to Janakamma.

Unfortunately, within a few years of his marriage, Basavaraja passed away. Mallasarja continued to inspire and support Chennamma and helped her deal with their son's death. She continued to look after their subjects.

Peshwa Bajirao II was a fugitive in those days. Despite that, he never missed an opportunity to attack smaller kingdoms. Around 1813, when he was in dire need of resources, he summoned Mallasarja to Edur, where he was camping.

'The Peshwa has called me to meet him at Edur,' Mallasarja told Chennamma.

'He will demand resources from you.'

'But we don't have much, Chenna. Guru Siddappa says he is annoyed with us for not paying him annual tributes.'

'I hope he understands how hard pressed we have been.'

'You take care of Kittur, I shall be back soon,' Mallasarja tried to assure his queen.

As expected, the Peshwa demanded a huge sum of money and troops from Mallasarja. He also forced Mallasarja to accept his subordination. When he refused, an annoyed Peshwa imprisoned him at Edur.

The news soon reached Kittur and Chennamma called upon Guru Siddappa to negotiate Mallasarja's release.

A lot of time passed, but Siddappa did not return, nor did he send any message to the Queen. Though she privately cried for her husband, Chennamma never neglected her duty towards the people of Kittur.

She sent a few more troops to Edur, but they too did not return.

Finally, in 1816, Mallasarja was released from the Marathas' captivity.

Seeing Siddappa coming back alone, the Queen cried out loud, 'Where is the King? How is he?'

'Mother, he fell seriously ill in the prison. A nervous Peshwa ordered his release.'

'Why did you not inform me about his illness?' Chennamma demanded.

'Mother, I was not allowed to return alone,' saying this, Siddappa began to sob. A worried Queen looked at the old noble.

'What happened?' she asked anxiously.

'Mother, Maharaj is no more. He died on the way.'

Meanwhile, the new governor-general of the East India Company, Hastings, had arrived in India with three very specific aims. The first was the hunting down of criminal Pindaries, the second was to bring the Marathas under the Company's subordination, and the third was the expansion of the British Empire. The Pindaries were even more dreadful than the dacoits. Horrible murders, indiscriminate loot, raping women and wanton destruction of villages were among their principal activities.

In the third war of Panipat, these criminals supported the Marathas. Since then, they have been hunting dogs for the Maratha rulers. By the time Baji Rao became the peshwa, the Pindaries had already established power over the Maratha territories south of River Narmada. Yet, the Peshwa continued patronizing them.

Now with Lord Hastings at the helm, the British and the Maratha clash was inevitable. In these circumstances, in 1816, Chennamma put her stepson Rudrasarja on the throne of Kittur.

In 1816, at Nagpur, Bhonsale of Barar was brought under the Company and by 1817, Hastings drove away the Pindaries beyond River Chambal. On 5 November 1817, Scindia was forced to enter into a shameful treaty at Kanpur. The British were now approaching Kirki faster to have the last fight with the Marathas.

Kittur's royal court deliberated upon the prevailing crisis.

'Queen, the Marathas have tormented us for long. This is the time to join the British and unite against them,' one influential nayaka, Mallappa advised.

'The Marathas are a spent force and the British will rule Hindustan. We should support them to save Kittur,' another nayaka, Venkata Rao, supported Mallappa.

'I also think so,' the young king Rudrasarja agreed to the proposal.

Chennamma opposed the idea.

'Rudra, I know the Marathas are your father's murderers. But, on no account should we help the foreigners against our own countrymen. Today, with our help, they will defeat the Marathas, and tomorrow, with someone else's help they will defeat us. This way, they will have won half of Hindustan.'

'What are you talking about? Do you think that if we support the Peshwa, he will feel obliged? No, I know their history very well. Please, don't stop me.'

Rudrasarja send Mallappa to inform the British that Kittur would fight along with them against the Peshwa. Thus, despite

Chennamma's disapproval, the soldiers of Kittur fought side by side with the Company.

In lieu of Kittur's help, the Company recognized Rudrasarja and his successors as the rulers of Kittur, on a payment of an annual tribute of rupees one lakh seventy thousand.

Chennamma was not happy.

'Son, this is the beginning of Kittur's fall.'

'Mother, you fail to understand that the treaty has brought us security. My successors and I will forever be the rulers of Kittur.'

'Son, that's true. But what about Kittur's independence?'

Rudrasarja chose not to reply. He failed to understand why his mother could not see the logic.

The difference in values of the mother and son created a chasm between the two. With that, the king came under the heavy influence of Mallappa and Venkata Rao. As a result, for the first time in its history, the Kittur army raided neighbouring states and sheltered vagabonds from other states.

Guru Siddappa and Chennamma tried to counsel Rudrasarja, but in vain.

The British collector of Dharwar saw a golden opportunity and began to interfere in the affairs of Kittur and warned Rudrasarja to not give shelter to the vagabonds and desist from troubling the neighbours.

As Veeramma, the wife of Rudrasarja, could not bear him an heir, Chennamma advocated for a second marriage, but Veeramma was against it.

Meanwhile, in 1824, Shivalinga Rudrasarja fell seriously ill.

'Kittur needs an heir, Mother,' seeing his imminent death, Rudrasarja cried.

'Son, have heart. You will soon be alright,' Chennamma could only say that much. In her heart, she knew that time was running out .

On 12 September 1824, a Sunday, Rudrasarja adopted a young boy Shivalingappa as his son on his deathbed. A letter was quickly drafted to send to Thackeray, the local British political agent, informing him of the adoption. The King managed to sign it a few moments before his death.

On the same day, a horse rider delivered the succession document to Thackeray, who dispatched Dr Bell to Kittur to treat the King. Dr Bell reached Kittur at night, and found that the King had already passed away.

Thackeray wanted to use the situation in the Company's favour. Under the policy of Paramountcy and Complete Authority (a precursor to the Doctrine of Lapse), without the prior approval of the Company, native rulers were not allowed to adopt a child, if they had no children of their own. In case their request was refused, the kingdom became a part of the Company automatically.

Thackeray decided to question the authenticity of the late king's letter.

After the death of Rudrasarja, Chennamma took the reins of the state in her hands. She wanted to groom young Shivalingappa, the way she had groomed her sons.

Chennamma's action was a big blow to Mallappa and Venkata Rao. They decided to set Thackeray against the Queen, and fixed a meeting with him in Kittur.

'Mallappa and Rao, you have been the closest friend to the late king. Tell me how he died.'

'He died of very high fever. Strange illness! Few days ago

he was perfectly healthy,' the shrewd Mallappa wove the net of suspicion.

'When did he die?'

'On Saturday....' Mallappa said cunningly and then looked at Venkata Rao to confirm.

'I am not sure. Perhaps it was a Sunday,' Rao's voice was unconvincing enough to influence Thackeray to make up his mind.

When Guru Siddappa called on Thackeray and tried to clarify the doubts, Thackeray volleyed him with a number of allegations.

'Guru, adoption without prior permission is invalid.'

'Collector, the illness was sudden and there was no time.'

'But, he died on Saturday, a day before the adoption.'

'That's a lie. The king died on Sunday, after the adoption.'

'No, he died before you could draft the letter.'

'That's a lie. There were witnesses.'

'All witnesses are your people. I know you all...,' he looked at Siddappa as if the old man was the main conspirator.

An angry Siddappa got up in protest and was about to leave, when Thackeray added insult to injury.

'Guru, I know, the pen with which one of you had signed was thrust into the fingers of a dead king.'

'This is outrageous. Take your despicable words back, Mr Collector,' Siddappa was now shaking with anger.

'I will be sending my conclusions to Commissioner Chaplin. Meanwhile, I will keep the law and order in my hands,' Thackeray announced.

'No one will accept that,' Siddappa said and stormed out of the camp.

Siddappa reported the entire discussion to Chennamma. An angry Queen put Mallappa and Venkata Rao to death for their treachery. She quickly summoned a meeting of the councillors. But, before they could gather, Thackeray marched into the fort with his soldiers and sealed the treasury.

His arrogance infuriated the people of Kittur. Rama Habshi, an African, and Sangolli Rayanna led the people to the palace. All the Africans living in Kittur came out to join Chennamma's army. They met Chennamma and expressed their solidarity.

'We cannot take this lying down,' the councillors shouted in unison.

'But, how can we fight the might of the Company?' Siddappa said. 'Tipu, the Mughals and even the powerful Marathas have been defeated by them.'

The Queen addressed her people in a firm voice. 'We are not letting them interfere in our affairs. We will fight for our rights. If we fear their might and not resist them today, then tomorrow they will suppress us more. How can we allow that?' She looked at Siddappa and then said, 'But all said and done, let us first try for a settlement. I shall write to Chaplin and, if needed, to Elphinstone as well.'

'No,' yelled an angry Rayanna. 'We will kill them all.'

'Let peace get a chance, Rayanna. Till the reply comes from Chaplin, I want you to stay calm.'

The people obeyed their Queen and returned with their hearts simmering.

Commissioner Chaplin refused to recognize Shivalingappa as the new ruler, and Chennamma as the regent. A disappointed Queen appealed before Governor Elphinstone at Bombay. But, he too turned down the request.

Immediately after the rejection of her appeal, Thackeray rode up to the fort with 200 men and four cannons of the Madras Native Horse Artillery. He placed the cannons in front of the main gate of the fort and asked his men to be ready for a coercive action. Satisfied with his preparations, and with an intention to confiscate the treasure and jewels of Kittur, valued around 15 lakh of rupees, he issued his warning to open the gate.

'The war has been thrust upon us, Guru Siddappa. Thackeray's arrogance has left us with no choice but to fight. Can a small village fight a mighty empire?'

'Queen Mother, we need your nod. My African friends and I will create havoc in the rank and files of the enemy. Order us to march,' Rama Habshi requested her.

'Why do you hesitate, Ma?' Guru Siddappa said, 'they have left us with no choice.'

The Queen went into her private chamber. After some time, the gates of her chamber flung opened and clad in white clothes, a fully armed Chennamma stood there, ready to lead them.

'Brave people of Kittur, let us fight and uphold the honour of our land. Independence is the most precious thing in the world. Today, the enemy will witness the might of our sword.'

'Ma, please go back to the palace. Let me lead the fight,' old Siddappa offered.

'I will lead my men, Guru Siddappa,' a smiling Queen moved her horse forward.

Like a torrent, Chennamma's soldiers gushed out and leapt on the enemy. Before the British cannons could boom,

Chennamma's sword cut the head of a British soldier. True to his promise, Rama Habshi created havoc within the British army and it ran helter skelter. Thackeray challenged his men and urged them to fight. Brandishing his sword, he moved ahead.

Chennamma's bodyguard Sayid Balappa saw him charging in and aimed his gun at the collector. Before Chennamma could stop him, Sayid shot him down and the brave soldiers of Kittur ran over the British army in a few minutes. Many British officers were taken prisoners.

Chennamma said a few words of caution to her cheering crowd.

'Friends, let us be more vigilant and better prepared for the endless struggle in the future.'

She sent her envoy to Kolhapur for help. But the Maratha chief proved to be a traitor. He handed over Kittur's envoy to the British.

Elphinstone got very angry on hearing about the severe blow to Company's prestige and he dispatched Chaplin from Pune to Belgaum. The British army also got replenishments from Bombay and Madras.

Despite a huge force under his command, Chaplin waited for his battery train to come. Huge cannons were moved through the marshy track between Belgaum and Kittur. Meanwhile, Chaplin bought time by negotiating with Chennamma's envoys.

'Let the Queen first set the British prisoners free. Then we can sit for the talks,' he sent a message to her.

'Ma, we should not release the prisoners. You cannot trust the treacherous Britons,' Siddappa advised her.

'I know that they cannot be trusted. But fighting a war on the strength of captives will be cowardice.'

'I heard Chaplin is just buying time. He will attack us once his battery train arrives.'

'I know that too. But, let us release the prisoners. Let us fight with dignity, valour and honour,' Chennamma was firm.

The Queen released all war prisoners. Two of the released officers, Walter Elliot and Senior Collector Stevenson urged Chaplin to stop the war.

'Sir, the Queen has behaved with dignity and look after us very well. She will be a great friend to us.'

Chaplin rejected their suggestions.

The British cannons opened fire and Chennamma's army again charged in on the enemy. A fierce battle began. Thomas Munro's nephew got killed in the war. Despite the blown up fort wall, Chennamma and her soldiers kept up an equal fight till a few treacherous sons of the soil mixed mud and cow dung in the gunpowder of Kittur's cannons.

The Kittur canons stopped firing. Chennamma, realizing the situation, tried to escape from the fort to regroup her men. Few British soldiers caught a glimpse of her and arrested her.

Before her capture, she gave the command of the freedom struggle in the hands of Sungolli Rayanna.

'Rayanna, this is not the end of the struggle. Keep the flag of freedom high and continue fighting the foreigners.'

Rayanna continued his guerilla war for freedom till 1829, until his capture. For five years, he remained a menace for British troops in the area. He wanted to install Shivalingappa on the throne of Kittur. A jealous nayaka, Linganna Shetty, who had wanted his own son to be adopted by Chennamma, treacherously got Rayanna captured by the British.

Rayanna was hanged in 1829, the same year when the brave queen of Kittur, Chennamma, died in prison in Bailhongal Fort.

They were about to reach home, when Moropant completed Chennamma's story.

'So, the Marathas betrayed Kittur twice,' Manu Bai commented and after a few seconds prophetically announced, 'when I become rani, I will ensure I take along everyone.'

'You and a rani?' Moropant laughed at his daughter's dream.

'Yes. One day I will be the rani.' Manu announced with determination.

Moropant was not aware then that Pundit Tatya Dikshit was waiting with a marriage proposal for Manu from Gangadhar Rao, the king of Jhansi.

Avantibai

'We are losing the battle, Your Highness,' Tatya Tope said in frustration.

'No, we are not! The Nawab of Banda with his strong cavalry of 2,000 and some infantry has joined us. We also have the best-drilled and organized rebel troops of Gwalior,' Rao Sahib rebuked Tatya.

'They are so unaware of reality,' Tatya thought in disgust, looking at the canopy in the far end. Tatya Tope was the most gifted leader that India had produced in the first war of independence. He was a remarkably learned youth with great planning and organizing capabilities, and an enthusiastic supporter of the home rule. Many scholars and commanders in the British camp considered him to be the mind behind the Indian mutiny and included him amongst the most famous guerilla leaders of the world.

Rao Sahib was the nephew of Nana Sahib, the rebel leader of Kanpur. After facing defeats on their home turf, the Rani of Jhansi, the Nawab of Banda, Rao Sahib and others had formed an allegiance to defend Kalpi and Gwalior.

It was a hot May night when the rebel leaders assembled to plan the future course of the war.

'Hugh Rose is accumulating a huge army at Putch. The next thirty days will be crucial. Who will win the war—the natives or the foreigners?' Nawab of Banda twisted his big moustache.

'Friends, Kalpi is just a small part in this long fight for independence. There are thousands of mutinies happening all over Hindustan. From Bengal to Punjab, from Himalayas to Narmada, people have risen up to drive out the feringhees. For the British, native states are just "petty intervening principalities" to be possessed. We have already lost most of our strongholds including Dilli, Kanpur, Lucknow and Jhansi.'

'But, the feringhees are only a few…' Rao Sahib tried to respond.

'Maharaj, you are wrong. They have a unified command and they move under a larger plan. They are organized and more than 350,000 in number. We may be more in number, but we are scattered. At a given point of time, we can hardly assemble a few hundred soldiers.

Now the British troops have arrived in Calcutta from Burma, Ceylon, Mauritius, Persia and England. I have heard that a few platoons have been moved even from Crimea. They have also diverted their troops from a military expedition on its way to China. To attack us, the king of Nepal has deployed a force of 9,000 Gurkhas from the hills.'

Tatya's information stunned everybody. No one spoke afterwards.

Later in the night, Lakshmi Bai called Tatya.

'Tatya, how can the Company* capture all the villages

---

*The East India Company ruled a large part of India from 1757 to 1858.

around the country? There is war everywhere.'

Tatya looked at Rani and then replied with a wry grin.

'Rani Sahib, so many small principalities and zamindars are fighting this war, but there is hardly any coordination,' Tatya paused. 'Sometimes, I feel proud of them, and yet pity them.'

'I don't get you.'

'You must have heard the inspiring prayer which talks of how Raja Shankar Shah had invoked a many-armed goddess to aid him to upset the British government. Our battles are like the limbs of the Raja's goddess. Rani Sahib, hundred arms are useful to fight and defeat a demon only if a visionary brain guides them. The distinct and conscious object of gaining freedom by destroying the British, inspires these mutinies. But, where is the central visionary leadership?'

Tatya waited for the Rani's response and then continued, 'Rani Sahib, when we attack first, we capture our forts and town. But for how long?' He looked at the Rani and then said, 'Only for a couple of months until a reinforced British army comes back to invade us. No one comes forward to support others. This is the story everywhere. You know what happened to Haji Imdadullah, Babu Kunwar Singh, Raja Shankar Shah, Begum Hazrat Mahal, Chimna Sahib, Khan Bahadur Khan, Mir Muhammad Hussain Khan, Avantibai and others?'

'Avantibai?' Lakshami Bai was unaware of this name.

'Yes, when she asked for assistance from the King of Rewa, he promised support, but later ditched her in face of crisis.'

'Tell me more about her,' Lakshmi Bai urged Tatya. 'Was she a queen? How have I never heard about her?'

Ramgarh is not a big state. It's a small village in Dinderi tehsil of Mandla in central Hindustan. Situated in the Mekala range of the Satpura mountains, the inhabitants of this area mostly belong to Gond and Baiga tribes.

Couple of centuries ago, Gaj Singh Lodhi formed this principality. There is an unconfirmed but popular tale about how the principality was formed. Once an unteamable man-eater had terrorized the villages of Gadha-Mandla. Two brothers from Ramgarh, Mohan Singh and Mukutmani, killed the tiger in a fierce fight, as a result of which, the younger brother, Mukutmani sustained heavy injuries and succumbed to them. A grateful king appointed the surviving brother, Mohan Singh, as his army chief. After the death of Mohan Singh, the king made his son, Gaj Singh, his vassal and gave him the Mukutpur region to overlook. Few months later, when the Gonds rebelled against the king of Gadha-Mandla, Gaj Singh suppressed them and killed their leaders. A pleased king added the Ramgarh estate to the vassalage of Gaj Singh and honoured him with the title of king.

A few years later, Gaj Singh declared his independence and expanded his kingdom to a few hundred villages. In 1780, the Marathas took Ramgarh under their control and when the British defeated them in 1818, they took it from the Marathas. Under a settlement reached in 1819–20, the estate was left with the king for a payment of Rs 2,000 per annum. The annual income of Ramgarh—with 442 populated villages—in those days amounted to about Rs 14,000.

Avantibai was born in the village of Mankeri in Narmada Valley. Her father Jujhar Singh was an ambitious zamindar in the Sivani district. He trained his daughter in horse riding, sword fighting and arranged for her education. She was a brave and beautiful girl. Jujhar Singh wanted to get his daughter married to some influential and powerful local Rajput prince and, hence, requested Raja Shankar Shah of Gadha-Mandla to mediate for his daughter's marriage proposal for Prince Vikramjit Singh, son of King Lachman Singh of Ramgarh. Lachman Singh accepted his proposal on the recommendation of Shankar Shah.

After a few weeks, on the auspicious day of Mahahivaratri, Avantibai and Vikramjit Singh got married. After the wedding, Avantibai found that her husband was of unsound mind, but she decided to take care of him. After sometime, she gave birth to a son, Aman Singh. In 1850, she gave birth to her second son, Sher Singh. Unfortunately, during that time, her father-in-law passed away, leaving the responsibility of Ramgarh and two young sons with her.

Taking advantage of the situation, the British took over the management of the estate and fixed a pension for Raja and his family.

Before Tatya could finish, Lakshmi Bai burst into anger. Her principality like many others was a victim of the Doctrine of Lapse and other Company tools used to annex Indian states. This was happening despite Indian kings and queens showing absolute loyalty to the British.

'Tatya, it is a shame that peace-loving kings and princes who had done no injury to the British, who like their ancestors, had been faithful to them, have been pushed aside. They were not cruel tyrants who butchered their people; neither did they neglect the welfare of their subjects. Then why did they thrust upon us that doctrine of lapse? Who are they to assume the role of a guardian angel in our motherland?'

Tatya said, 'Rani Sahib, the same thing happened in Ramgarh. After the death of Lachman Singh, Avantibai ruled the kingdom in the name of both Vikramjit Singh and Aman Singh. In 1851, the British combined Mandla, Sohagpur and Ramgarh and made a new district under Sagar division. Avantibai did not like it and protested, but in vain. Jabalpur was the headquarters of Sagar division under Major W.C. Erskine, who was also the commissioner, and Ramgarh was made a subdivision. Mandla was governed by a collector, Captain H.F. Waddington. As Mandla was yet to have a collector's bungalow, Waddington used to spend the summer and monsoon months in Jabalpur.'

'I remember, you and the Maulvi Sahib were in touch with Raja Shankar Shah of Gadha-Mandla,' Lakshmi Bai knew that the Raja was chosen to lead the revolt in central Hindustan.

'We started sending chapatis to Gadha and the Jabalpur area from January 1857. Our volunteers were active in the area. Stories about the British's deliberate mixing of pig fat, cow blood and bone powder in ghee, wheat flour and sugar were widespread. People were convinced that the Company was hell-bent on polluting their faith.'

On Nana Sahib's advice, Raja Shankar Shah charted a secret plan. The native soldiers of 52 Regiment, Shankar Shah's son Raghunath Shah, Raja Saraju Prasad of Vijayraghavgarh, Thakur Jagat Singh, the revenue collector of Shahpur and many local zamindars were party to it. That was the time when Avantibai gave birth to her third son. But the responsibilities of maternity could not stop her in actively joining the plan. She encouraged many zamindars of her region, such as Garul Singh of Sohagpur, Balbhadra Singh of Kothi Nigwani, Vijay Singh of Shahpur, and Khuman Singh of Mukas, to fight against the British.

Avantibai wrote poems to inspire her people. She used to send messengers to the neighbouring states, with her poems and bangles. One of her popular poems was:

> देश और आन के लिए मर मिटो, या फिर चूड़ियाँ पहनों।
> तुम्हें धर्म और ईमान की सौगन्ध, जो इस कागज का पता दुश्मन को दो।
>
> *(Raise your sword,*
> *To die for honour of your country*
> *Else wear bangles.*
> *Swore by your faith,*
> *You invite His wrath,*
> *If you ever disclose this plan to the foe.)*

'This is the second month of the monsoons, we should attack the cantonment before Muharrum,' Avantibai proposed in the meeting.

'We will begin from Jabalpur, Rani Sahib. You wait for our signal,' Raja Shankar Shah advised her.

'I shall be visiting all the local landlords and the kings. I am sure by Ashwin, we will assemble more than 5,000 men.'

'That will be sufficient for Erskine. Once we defeat him, Rani Sahib can control Waddington,' Raghunath Shah, son of

Shankar Shah, was an enthusiastic youth.

'We should do it simultaneously, everywhere. In Mandla, the Company has only 100 soldiers, and in Ramgarh, Waddington has 120 soldiers and twenty horses,' Avantibai informed them.

'No. We should not divide our power. Further, in Mandla and Ramgarh, majority of the Company soldiers are natives.'

Avantibai did not like the idea but kept quiet. Raghunath Shah and others charted out a grand plan to assemble soldiers from all over the region.

Somehow, Commissioner Erskine got a whiff of the plan. The rebel leaders could not see beyond their local and selfish interests. Therefore, they were not cautious enough to guard their joint interests. Girdharidas, a petty zamindar, spilled the beans and the British Commissioner at Jabalpur got the hint.

Erskine sent his peon in disguise of a faqir to Raja Shankar Shah. It was famously said that no one had ever returned from the Raja's palace empty handed. Erskine's peon reached the palace in guise of a faqir who could see the future. When the peon began telling the old king about his past, the king was so impressed that he asked the most pertinent question of his life to the fraudulent faqir.

'When will these feringhees leave our land?'

The faqir closed his eyes and meditated for a long time. Without opening his eyes, he spoke as if in a trance.

'It is possible, Raja. But, you have to ensure an auspicious time, day, and alliance.'

To confirm the perfect planetary combination, the old and naïve Raja said everything to that unknown faqir.

That night, the faqir returned to the palace with Lieutenant

Clark and about fifty Company soldiers. Raja, his son and thirteen other members of his family were arrested from his palace. Raja's property was confiscated and a thorough search ended with Clark finding a piece of paper on which a prayer was written, urging the many-armed goddess to wipe out the British. The Raja and his family were charged for treason in a public trial and were found guilty. After a few days, they were publicly assassinated.

Shankar Shah's death created palpable tension in the region. Agitated zamindars and peasants requested Avantibai to lead them, while the infuriated people were impatient and attacked the tehsil and police post of Shahpura. Few government officials were killed and government buildings were torched. Sensing that the British would retaliate, Avantibai quickly sent assistance to the zamindar of Shahpur, Vijay Singh. Avantibai captured Ramgarh and planned to march towards Mandla with Vijay Singh and Garul Singh of Sohagpur.

Around that time, the natives of 52 Regiment at Jabalpur rebelled. This was quickly followed by revolts in Patan and Salminabad cantonments.

Avantibai's call for rebellion aroused a powerful wave of revolution. Led by her and the ruler of Vijayraghavgarh, Saraju Prasad, the entire Mandla region joined hands for an armed rebellion.

'Ramgarh is virtually ruled by the Queen. The King is no more than her pawn. I am keeping a tab on the Queen's brother Seetaram, her chief minister Sukayee and his son. Kindly provide a troop of Madras Native Infantry to keep control over Mandla. If the rebels get Mandla, it will create a lot of inconvenience for us,' Waddington wrote to Erskine.

Waddington knew very well that till Mandla was with the British, it was difficult for Avantibai to get Sivni. Avantibai sent a platoon of rebels to the hills between Ramnagar and Ghughri forcing the government officials to quickly desert Ramnagar. A worried Waddington sent twenty-five riflemen to Ghughri and recaptured Ramnagar. In retaliation, her soldiers seized Jabalpur Road, thus, effectively blocking all communication between Mandla and Jabalpur.

'Sahib, we should leave this place,' a subdivisional officer urged Waddington.

'No. My priority is to restore communication between Mandla and Jabalpur. After that, I will get Ramgarh.'

Watching an unconvinced tehsildar, Waddington assured him, 'I am writing to get help from Sivni. But, I have one more idea. These Gonds are very loyal to Avantibai. I will break this alliance,' Waddington smiled wickedly and explained his strategy to his officers.

For the next three days, Waddington toured nearby tribal areas and tried to rally the Gonds to not support Avantibai. When he saw that the people remained unconvinced, he terrorized the Queen's supporters by hanging five Gonds to death, on charge of treason.

As a result, about 200 workers of Avantibai left their posts at Ramgarh.

This setback prompted the Queen to take some immediate measures to restore people's confidence in her. After her persuasion, the Gond chief of Imalae joined her army. With her 2,000 strong soldiers, a confident Rani attacked the village of Kheri, a little away from Mandla. Waddington decided to wait and watch. An entire night he kept a vigil on eastern roads. In the morning, he got information of the advance of a platoon of rebels from Jabalpur coming to assist Avantibai. Keeping a handful of soldiers with him, Waddington ordered his remaining force to attack the rebels; 400 rebels were up against 60 soldiers of Waddington. However, the careless rebels could not endure a sudden attack and lost. As a result, 21 rebels were captured and promptly hanged on nearby trees.

After consolidating her position at Kheri, Avantibai intended to invade Mandla. But before she could do that, a confident Waddington arrived at Kheri to suppress the rebellion. Avantibai and Waddington, riding on their horses, led their troops and attacked each other. At one moment, the two came face to face. Avantibai's sword was flashing like a lightning and she struck Waddington with her sword. Waddington lunged his horse and ducked. The horse moved a step forward and the sword hit it with great force; the injured horse fell on the ground, and Waddington jumped off his horse and escaped.

Avantibai sent a few platoons to the south and northwest of Mandla, and encouraged the defeated rebels of Jabalpur to return. The news of Mandla's siege stirred the natives in Waddington's army.

'I need to go to Sivni to get reinforcements,' Waddington told his tehsildar.

The tehsildar's glance was enough to communicate his discomfort.

'You shall not leave Mandla till I return with reinforcement. Got it?' Waddington reiterated.

The tehsildar did not utter a word.

'OK. When you feel that it is not possible to defend Mandla, then come to Sivni with prisoners, treasury and records.'

The tehsildar quit Mandla immediately after Waddington left. By the evening, Avantibai had control over almost the entire Mandla district.

For the next two months, Avantibai ruled over Mandla.

Captain Waddington did not sulk in silence after his humiliating departure from Mandla. Erskine sent Lieutenant Burton and Lieutenant Cockburn with the Nagpur Irregulars and 52 Native Infantry with him. First, Sohagpur and then Narayanganj, Patan, Salminabad and Babeha were snatched from the hands of the rebels. Avantibai attacked Ahmadpur and Anjania. Meanwhile, Waddington consolidated his position at Mandla and nearby areas. The Rani sent a platoon to capture an important village Binaika, near Mandla, but it failed badly.

A disappointed Avantibai retreated to Ramgarh.

'The British are inching closer to us. We need external assistance to survive. You should speak to the Raja of Rewa,' Vijay Singh advised Avantibai.

'Many Brahmins and Rajputs from village Chandia of Rewa have joined us. Few months back, the Maharaja agreed to help us in crisis. I will send an envoy to him,' Avantibai welcomed the proposal.

Bolstered by the reinforcement, Waddington won Ghughry without resistance and planned to capture Ramgarh. He attacked Ramgarh from two sides—Burton and Cockburn attacked from one side, while Waddington charged from the other side.

Avantibai had sensed that she was not in a position to resist the strength of the British army. She quickly decided to vacate Ramgarh, and continue her fight from the forests of Devhargarh hills.

When Waddington reached Ramgarh, he found it deserted. Waddington occupied the royal residence and made it his headquarters.

In the hills of Devhargarh, the Queen reassembled her scattered army. Her infant son died in the jungle due to the hardship but she was spared no time to mourn.

'Rani Sahib, Cockburn will rule from the Ramgarh palace. Waddington is planning to win Shahpur and Sohagpur,' Vijay Singh informed Avantibai.

'Garul Singh has not returned from Rewa. Do you think King Jagannath will keep his promise?' Aman Singh asked.

'No,' the Queen said. 'Our envoy led by Garul Singh was imprisoned by the King. He has somehow managed to escape from Rewa, but the King has sent six cannons for Waddington. I don't think we will get any external help. We are running short of ration and ammunition.'

Hopes of help were now shattered. The rainy season was about to begin and the Queen looked at her dispirited men and then announced, 'Brave soldiers, Bhagwan Shri Krishna has said that the soul is immortal and indestructible. No one is able to destroy that imperishable soul. This material body will come to end, if not today, then tomorrow for sure. Therefore, fight. Fighting for our motherland is our prime duty; why should there be any hesitation?' The Queen paused and then took out her sword from the scabbard and flashed it in the air.

'My brave men, only fortunate men get an opportunity to fight for their motherland. If today, we shun our duty, this sin will destroy our reputation forever. And know it well, that dishonour is worse than death. Bhagwan says, either you will be killed on the battleground and attain heaven, or you will conquer and enjoy the earthly kingdom. Therefore, get up with determination and fight.'

Avantibai divided her troops into three parts and marched down the hill. The air filled with war cries and flashing swords, her soldiers came out in the open. The sword flashing rebels were within the range of the British rifles. Waddington, seeing the golden opportunity, ordered to shoot the rebels from both the sides.

Determined to fight, Rani's valiant soldiers kept falling down but never stopped marching ahead.

Very soon, Burton also joined Waddington and surrounded the rebels from three sides. A bloody battle resumed in the lanes of Ramgarh; an uneven fight between sword and gun was on. Ignoring the approaching bullet, the brave soldiers of Avantibai were fighting their way through the enemy force to make their way up to the palace. Their attack was so fierce that Waddington had to retreat. But before the rebels could take over the palace, forces of some northern states and Rewa arrived to help the British.

In a few moments, the war scene changed. The enemies were now surrounding the Queen and in no time, she was left with only a handful of soldiers. Flashing her sword and galloping on her horse, she moved out of Ramgarh. Burton and Waddington chased her for many miles until she disappeared into the hills.

'Time is running out,' she called her trusted man Mahipal Singh. 'You, Aman Singh, Vijay Singh and Bahadur Singh should go to Sohagpur. Waddington will go there. That fort is now our only hope. That fort cannot be taken over without cannons. We should make that our headquarters,' Rani looked at the direction of the noise. The enemies were closing in.

'Mahipal, tell everyone that I shall lead them from the hills. Give them my blessings. Now, move fast.'

Once Mahipal departed, only four men were left with her. She called the senior soldier, Umrao Singh.

'Umrao, the enemy would like to capture me alive. I would rather die than allow them to arrest me. I am moving inside the caves. You three, stop them here.'

'Rani Sahib, let them witness the mettle of my sword. Until I am alive, no one will reach near you.'

The British soldiers were very close when Umaro Singh jumped on them like death incarnate and slaughtered many of them. But, the enemy troops were swarming like locusts.

From the insides of her cave, the Queen saw the fall of her men. The dream to liberate Ramgarh was shattered. Her position was extremely precarious and her capture now was imminent.

She remembered her ancestor, Durgavati. 'Falling into the unholy hands of feringees will be a disgrace.' She made a firm decision and jumped off her horse and drove it away. All alone, in the midst of defeat and her men's death, the Queen plunged her own sword into her belly and died.

For a long time, no one spoke. Lakshami Bai thought long and then said with emotion dripping in her voice:

'Tatya, I am not disheartened. These sacrifices may not give us freedom today. But, I am sure that tomorrow their stories will inspire millions of Indians to find a way to freedom. This is not failure. We are fighting Enfield Rifles with swords and spears. I remember once Nana had said, "These blue-capped rifles kill even before the trigger is pulled".'

Tatya looked at the Rani's face but there was no sign of fatigue on it.

'Tatya, they have the services of Bombay, Madras and Deccan. Sindh, Rajasthan, Nepal and Afghanistan too are with them. Their resources are endless and they are armed with the most destructive and latest weaponry. They have electric telegraph lines to communicate. We are hardly organized. All of us have different goals except our hatred for foreigners. Apart from Maulvi Sahib and you, perhaps, no one has any connection with the rebels fighting in different regions.'

Rani raised the glow of the lamp. 'I am not disheartened. Let us make Gwalior the seat of rebellion. Let us begin from this nucleus. Scindia has remained loyal to the feringhees, but we now have the fort of Gwalior to begin the second phase of war.'

Tatya bowed and took leave of the Rani to prepare for next day's war.

Lakshmi Bai

Sharp eyed and stylish, John Lang was reputed to be a unique travel writer and diarist in north India, during the troubled times of mutiny.

His mind was obsessing over Jhansi since morning, when his messenger, Badaru, brought him the news of the Rani's death.

Lang remained stunned for a few moments. Exactly four years ago, Lakshmi Bai, the queen of Jhansi, had gifted him an elephant, an expensive Arab camel, a pair of greyhounds, Jhansi's silks and a pair of shawls to plead her case with the directors of the Company.

Lang remembered his inappropriate remark when, by a stroke of chance, he happened to have a glimpse of the Rani. Just for a brief moment, the Rani's adopted child had unknowingly drawn the curtain aside, and Lang saw her for the first time.

The Rani was very young. Her round face was the epitome of beauty with fine eyes and a delicately shaped nose. Wearing no ornaments, except for a pair of gold earrings, and in a plain white muslin sari, she had a remarkably fine figure chiselled through years of discipline and hard outdoor exercises. Her smile was disarming. The Rani had asked him to help her in her case against the confiscation of her estate and the refusal of the governor-general to accept Damodar Rao, her adopted son, as the legal heir of Jhansi.

Taken aback with her beauty, Lang had remarked, 'If Dalhousie could only be as fortunate as I have been, he would have at once given Jhansi back to its beautiful queen.'

The Queen had overlooked Lang's unseemly compliment and had asked him to pursue her case.

'It won't be of any use.' John Lang had said, 'Now, the governor-general cannot restore Jhansi to your son.'

'Then?'

'You have to appeal to the queen in England. I will help you in writing a petition. Meanwhile, you keep on drawing the pension.'

'I will not give up my Jhansi,' the Queen had exclaimed.

'Rani Sahib, it will be futile to fight the British. Captain Gorden's army is here. Any action could destroy the faint hope of getting Jhansi restored.'

'Gentleman, people of Jhansi will not accept the Company's rule.'

Despite Lang's best persuasion, the Queen would not consent to draw any pension from the British.

That was the first and final meeting John Lang had with the Rani of Jhansi. But since then, never for a day, he could forget her grit, generosity and character. Even in her lifetime the Rani, as her allies and enemies called her, had become a phenomenon.

After the conclusive defeat of the Marathas in the third Anglo-Maratha war and by the treaty of 1818, a victorious East India Company deprived the last Maratha Peshwa Baji Rao of his dominions and exiled him to Bithur, near Kanpur, to live a quiet life with a pension of Rs 800,000. Lakshmi Bai's father, Moropant, was in the service of Peshwa.

In the absence of a biological son, the exiled Peshwa Baji Rao adopted Dhundhu Pant—or Nana Sahib as he came to be known later—as his son. Nana Sahib and Lakshmi Bai had grown up together at Bithur.

Manu Bai, as Lakshmi Bai was called before her marriage, was trained in horse riding and warfare with Nana Sahib and his brother. At a young age, she was married to the much older king of Jhansi, Gangadhar Rao. After the wedding, she was named Lakshmi Bai. She exhibited an extraordinary balance in pursuing her outdoor hobbies as well as managing the affairs of the state. In fact, she pioneered women education in Jhansi and also started regimenting women as warriors.

In Bithur, Peshwa Baji Rao lived a quiet life till his death in 1851. After his death, the government permitted Nana Sahib to inherit the savings of Baji Rao, but refused to grant him the title of Peshwa as well as the pension. Nana, then, appealed in a logical and convincing manner to the court of directors against the decision of the governor-general. He even cited examples of Delhi and Mysore and asked them not to differentiate between him and other native princes, but his appeal was rejected in May 1853.

Lakshmi Bai was going through a similar predicament. The king of Jhansi had been particularly faithful to the British. In fact, Lord William Bentinck had presented the then king of Jhansi a British ensign and a letter giving him the title of Raja, and had assured him that the title and the independence attached to it would be guaranteed by the British Government to him, his heirs and successors, including those who were adopted.

In 1851, Lakshmi Bai gave birth to a son who, unfortunately, died in infancy. The King could not recover from the loss and died in 1852. Before his death, he adopted a five-year-old child Damodar Rao as his heir in a public ceremony attended by the local British resident.

Lord Dalhousie refused to grant the right of adoption to the widowed Lakshmi Bai and declared that Jhansi had lapsed to the paramount power. Without the slightest shadow of pretence, he annexed Jhansi on 27 February 1854. Despite the Rani's many requests with evidences of the past, Dalhousie remained unmoved. He knew the might of his legions as compared to Rani's meagre force of 1,000 horsemen. The annual revenue of Jhansi at that time was Rs 600,000. Dalhousie fixed a pension for Rani at Rs 60,000 per annum.

The Rani tried to annul or reverse the order of annexation, but in vain. On 2 August 1854, the directors of the Company deprived the high-spirited queen of her genuine rights. The order converted the Queen, a character deeply respected, into an enemy of the British Company.

That was the time when the Rani called John Lang in a faint hope of pleading her case successfully before the board of directors. Though John had failed in his mission he had since kept in contact with people of Jhansi. If he knew someone had recently visited Jhansi, Lang often used to ask about the Queen and her Jhansi.

From the visitors' account, the year 1856 looked ordinary on the surface but there was turbulence foaming underneath.

It was the night of Diwali in 1856. After prayers and offerings Lakshmi Bai came into her drawing hall where Tatya Tope and Nana Sahib were waiting for her.

'Manu, Maulavi Ahmadullah and I have discussed the entire plan. The ground is ripe and people are ready to throw away the burden of the Company from their shoulders,' Nana Sahib told her.

'How can you be so optimistic?'

'Rani Sahib, the land reforms introduced by Thomson in the north-west provinces have prompted the people there to revolt,' Tatya explained. 'People are ready to fight for their rights. Since the beginning of the Burmese war, despite the promise of only making them serve on land, the soldiers are being sent across the sea. When many sipahis and their commanding officers refused, Dalhousie arbitrarily selected a regiment stationed at Barrackpur and sent it to foreign lands. Sipahis knew that touching the seawater would pollute their dharma, so they flatly refused to embark. The new governor, Canning, has now passed a law that everyone has to be available to serve across the seas.'

'Rani Sahib, sipahis are the back bone of company's rule and now they mistrust it.' Nana added.

'What about the rulers of various riyasats ?' Rani asked.

'It is sad,' Tatya looked at Rani. 'The Sikhs, Scindia and many others are happy with the Company. I see no revolt in South India either. The Company is too big to be won by small kingdoms and zamindars. Only a united power of the people can defeat it.'

'How can ordinary people fight the most modern army of the Company?'

'The way you are fighting, Rani Sahib. By training people, by inspiring them, by inducting them in your army,' Tatya replied without hesitation.

'The sipahis from Awadh region possess the right of petitioning the British resident at the Court of Lucknow on all matters affecting their own interests, and the interests of their family in their area. Do you know how big a privilege this is?'

The Rani nodded in agreement. 'If the resident of Lucknow advocates the personal affairs of a sipahi in the court of a native judge, it is obvious who wins.'

'Yes!' Tatya exclaimed. 'The advantage of possessing such a powerful advocate is so great that Awadh has become the Company's best recruiting ground in India. As a result, 90 per cent of the Bengal army is from Awadh.'

'If it is so, then it goes against our interest.'

'Not now.' Tatya smiled. 'This right of petition has now been abolished after the annexation of Awadh. This annexation is felt as a personal loss by every sipahi because it has deprived them of an ancient privilege. With the disappearance of this privilege, the sipahis have lost their standing in the society.'

Tatya took a pause and then continued, 'And the peasants are suffering too. The very nature of the Company is such that it interferes with every constituent of the Indian way of living. At every step, it disregards and humiliates our existence. Our artisans and weavers are dying as the Company forces us to use foreign machine-made goods. The farmers are forced to sell their produce for nothing. I have discussed it with Nazim Mohammad Hussain in Gorakhpur, Kunvar Singh and Amar Singh in Bhojpur, and they all agree that the time has come.'

'Who will initiate it?' Lakshmi Bai asked.

'Maulavi Ahmadullah has planned it. We can defeat them only when from Sindh to Assam, from Awadh to Madras, every sipahi and every farmer strikes at the same time, on the same day.'

'Impossible. Do you think such secret and vast communication is possible?'

'We will invite everyone, like we do on auspicious occasions,' Tatya smiled. 'The chapati will be our secret sign. The circulation of chapatis will notify them that a great rising is about to take place on the first favourable opportunity, and it will not raise any suspicion either as it is common and easy to pass on,' Tatya explained.

'The Company soldiers get handsome perks and privileges. Why will they take up arms against such an employer?'

'I think you are asking about an instrument which can trigger the rebellion,' Tatya said. 'Maulvi Ahmadullah had toured various battalions extensively and has discovered the instrument which should explode the already excited minds of the sipahis.'

Lakshmi Bai was now curious to know the entire plan.

'Few months back, the governor-general had authorized the production and introduction of a new cartridge, the exterior of which is smeared with fat. This fat is either pig or cow fat. This greasing is a well-thought out scheme to deprive the Hindus of their caste and to degrade the Muslims.'

'When will they start using these greased cartridges?' Lakshmi Bai asked.

'From January 1857. The moment they start using it in Calcutta, Maulvi Sahib will spread the news in all regiments. It will take three to four months.'

'What about the money, ammunitions and arms?' Rani asked.

'We have collected enough,' Tatya replied. 'Begum Hazrat Mahal in Lucknow and Begum Zeenat Mahal in Delhi have agreed. If everyone agrees, then let it begin at 11 am on 31 May 1857.'

'How will the sipahis keep patience for five months? And how will they know when is the right time to strike?'

'The lotus begins to bloom from April. We will tell the leaders to restrain the sipahis till a lotus flower appears in the barracks of the cantonment,' Tatya had the reply ready.

'If so, let us all begin tirthyatras to make people aware,' Rani suggested.

'Maulvi Sahib will start circulating pamphlets from January,' Tatya concluded the meeting.

'Badaru, this much only I knew from my sources. Tell me, what happened after that meeting? Jhansi was one of the last districts where rebellion spurted. What was in her mind?' Lang asked his messenger Badaru.

'Sahib, the Rani was determined to follow the agreed date of rebellion. I had seen how she had transformed the women of Jhansi.' Badaru replied.

'Badaru, I know she regimented the women of Jhansi. In the entire country, Jhansi is the only place where they have women platoons, companies and battalion.'

'Not only that Sahib. In Jhansi's army the number of Maharastrian women was very less. The majority of women were from Bundelkhand, that too from all castes and social strata. Only the Rani could do such miracle. It was an awe-inspiring sight for visitors from outside seeing women of Jhansi walking in market place and temples without purdah. They say the Rani has already freed the spirit of Bundelkhandi women.'*

This description brought tears into the eyes of John Lang.

'Badaru, I will tell you something that happened before my eyes. The Rani was a master cavalier and had a great eye for quality horses. One day, a trader had brought two identical looking horses in the durbar. Both horses were white, tall and healthy.

"How much for them?" the Rani had asked.

"One thousand for each, Your Highness." The trader had admiringly looked at his horses.

"I would like to examine both." The Rani had said and asked her commander to take the animals to the ground.

When she returned after an hour, she told the trader, "I will pay thousand for the first but only fifty for the second."

'Curious courtiers looked at each other. The trader thought

---

*Lakshmi Bai was a Maratha. Despite being a non-upper caste, in later centuries, the Maratha warrior class almost evolved into a higher caste themselves. They looked down on the locals, that is, the Bundelkhandis. The Marathas held the higher posts in state administration and court. In such an environment, Lakshmi Bai encouraged the Bundelkhandis and gave them more positions in the army and administration without any social bias.

for a while and then politely asked the Rani, "Rani Sahiba, why thousand for one and only fifty for the other?"

"The second horse has a longstanding internal injury near the chest."

'In a stunned court, the trader did accept the fact and apologized.'

Both remained silent for a long time.

'Badaru, tell me how Jhansi fought her war for freedom.'

It was past midnight. Millions of stars were twinkling in the cold and dark night. The Queen, wide awake, was still rocking on an armchair planning for the future. Thousands of letters had been circulated among the Indian soldiers of British East India Company urging them to raise arms against their British masters. Everything was going as planned till the news of the unplanned rebellion of Mangal Pandey disturbed the plans of a unified rebellion.

At Dumdum, on 15 January, a thirsty lascar working in the factory asked a Brahmin sipahi of Barrackpur to let him have a drink from his pot. The high-caste sipahi refused. The lascar in reply taunted the Brahmin, 'Don't worry. Soon, we all will be the same when we have to bite cartridges smeared with the fat of the cow and the pig.'

The story spread like wildfire. On 26 January, the telegraph house at Barrackpur was burnt and the sipahis of 19 Native Infantry refused to use the new cartridges. Leaders tried to calm the agitated soldiers and advised them to wait till 31 May. British commanders tried to suppress the growing rebellion in the battalion by using forceful measures but one high-caste sipahi, Mangal Pandey, lost his patience and killed a few British officers. Later on, the British hanged him.

This news of the incident spread everywhere and even the soldiers in the British barracks at Jhansi were itching to raise arms.

'What should I do? Start the rebellion or wait for the agreed date?' the Rani thought hard and decided to wait till the confirmed date.

Next day, the Company's representative, Deputy Commissioner Garden, visited her.

'Your Highness, promise to help us in case matters get worse.'

'Mr Garden, we have neither soldiers nor the required ammunition. Jhansi has been an ally of the British. If the Company agrees, I can strengthen my army,' the Rani sensed an opportunity.

Garden agreed. The Rani immediately started inducting youth in her army.

Unfortunately, Meerut too erupted in rebellion before time. On 6 May 1857, native sepoys killed some British soldiers and marched towards Delhi. Thereafter, they declared Bahadur Shah Zafar as the emperor of India, thereby sparking the rebellion all over North India much before the agreed date.

On June 4, one havildar of 12 Native Infantry captured the Star Fort at Jhansi and assembled Indian soldiers there. They killed a few British officers and torched the Company records. The Rani tried to save the British women and children but the rebels killed all of them. When the Rani refused to join them, the rebels went to Jalaun, Urai and then reached Kanpur.

The British refused to believe the Rani's innocence and

accused her of the carnage.

She called for a conference of all her people. The support she received from the people of Jhansi was overwhelming and soon the district was declared an independent state.

The Queen started recruiting for the army, in order to face the upcoming British challenge. But even before the British, the enemies within her kingdom challenged her.

A distant nephew of her late husband, Sadashiv Rao, claimed his right over Jhansi and rebelled. The Rani, in a swift response, defeated him. Similarly, the invasions of the neighbourhood principalities of Datia and Orchha were also neutralized.

A grand durbar was held to celebrate the victory. The Rani deliberated with guests about carrying forward the war of independence. By now, Zafar and Nana Sahib had been defeated in Delhi and Kanpur, respectively.

'Will it be Jhansi's turn next?' Nana Bhopatkar, her chief advisor, was worried.

'No. Jhansi never admits defeat. Jhansi kee jo latee takai, tihin khayen kalka mai.'* Lakshmi Bai directed them to accelerate the preparations.

Storing adequate food and fodder, and recruiting women troops, nursing staff and women gunners were her quick initiatives. Her inspiring leadership encouraged hundreds of women to join various departments of the government. She herself supervised their training and progress.

On 17 December 1857, Hugh Rose arrived to take the

---

*If someone dares to look at Jhansi, Goddess Durga will destroy him. This is a line from a famous poem written by a local goldsmith Bhaggi Dauju.

command of two brigades deployed in Central India. A diplomat by training, he was a veteran of Syrian, Turkish and Crimean wars. The governor-general put a huge force under his command.

He marched quickly towards Jhansi.

Winning Sahor, Rahatgarh, Banpur, Sagar, Garhakota, Narhat, Surahi, Maraura and Tal-Bahat, he marched towards Jhansi.

To support him, Brigadier Stuart was sent when Rose was barely 17 miles away from Jhansi.

Badaru could see tears in the eyes of his master.

'Badaru, how could she face the dreaded Hugh Rose for two months with her meagre resources?' John Lang wiped his tears.

'Sahib, when Rose was planning to attack Jhansi, Tatya Tope and his 900 followers had seized Charkhari. His win inspired six regiments of the Gwalior contingent and many locals to join him. Within a week, his army swelled to 22,000 men and 28 guns. He marched to Jhansi to help Lakshmi Bai.'

'Rose reached Jhansi on 21 March,' Badaru continued. 'The moment he saw the fort, Rose got awestruck by its strength.'

'I have not seen such a formidable fort in Central India,' Hugh Rose commented in admiration. 'Stuart, with that elevated rock, they don't need a huge brick base. Look at the work of masonry—there are guns peeping from every elevation. The Queen's fame is not exaggerated.'

'Sir, the city is four and a half miles in circumference and is built on a rock on three sides. The fourth side is the rock itself. The walls are six to eight feet thick and thirteen to eighteen feet high, having countless flanking bastions armed as batteries,' Stuart informed his boss.

'Yes, a fort garrisoned by 11,000 men, commanded by a woman who possesses all the instincts, courage and resolutions of a warrior,' Rose said removing his telescope.

When they were taking a reconnaissance, an old Muslim spy was brought before them.

'Sir, I am Peer Ali, a servant of Nawab Ali Bahadur. Nawab Sahib is a well-wisher of the company. He offers his assistance to you in all possible ways. We will help you from inside the fort.'

Rose happily accepted the help and attacked the fort in the night of 22 March 1858.

For nine days, Rose continuously fired shots and shells on the fort. But, Jhansi's women handled the defence and repaired the walls.

The women and children were assisting in the repair of the damage done by Rose's army, nursing the injured and carrying food and water to the soldiers on duty.

'Call Peer Ali, we need his master's help,' a frustrated Rose demanded.

At the same time, he got the news that Tatya Tope was advancing to Jhansi to help the queen.

'Let us go and stop him,' Stuart suggested.

'No. Any interruption to sieging operations would give the Rani the confidence to inspire and command her people. I want to crush her confidence.'

'How?'

'I will send only one-third of my men to counter Tatya. They will hide on both sides of the road at night. Early in the morning, when Tatya's army would be sluggish and arrive within our striking range, we will open fire. He will then have to face our infantry from the front.'

The sudden and powerful three-pronged attack, delivered with perfect precision, surprised Tatya's army; his first line broke and fled.

'If I could save my men and my guns, I could wage the war again,' Tatya retreated with that determination.

This defeat had an unfortunate effect. The Gwalior contingent of Tatya's army was not motivated enough anymore and they all surrendered before the British.

News of Tatya's defeat demoralized Jhansi, and Rose resolved to take advantage of the situation. He attacked the fort early next morning, and a desperate fight began. The British had tremendous difficulties in reaching the fort—the rampart was too high to scale. At that moment, someone opened the fort gates and the attackers marched into the palace. Despite this treachery, the Rani and his army put a highly spirited and stubborn fight that continued for the whole day and night.

When the invading army approached, the Rani took advantage of the darkness and disorder, and slipped out in disguise with trusted followers and rode to Kalpi. More than 5,000 fighters of Jhansi were killed that day against 343 invaders.

Rose reassembled his army and chased the fighters. Huge's army, reinforced by Rajput companies, splattered all the ravines and pathways leading to Gwalior.

On 16 June, Sir Huge and General Robert Napier attacked the rebels at Morar and completely surrounded them. The next morning, the Rajput army under General Smith attacked the Rani's force on a hilly ground between Kotha-ki-Sarai and Gwalior. The moment Smith's army arrived, Rani Lakshmi Bai ordered her cannons to fire. Smith cleverly pulled his army back and allowed the Queen to march ahead. When the Rani's army slackened a bit, Smith attacked her from all directions.

The Queen analyzed the situation in a flash and attacked the rear wing of the Rajput army forcing them within the range of her cannons. With less than a hundred soldiers, she fought valiantly and forced Smith to retreat.

Huge Rose understood that the position taken up by Smith had left him exposed to the Rani's attack. He resolved to kill the Rani. On 18 June, early in the morning, the Rani heard the British bugle and then the boom of their cannons.

'Deshmukh, I am leaving Damodar with you. If I get killed, take him away safely,' She told her assistant and held the hand of her adopted son for the last time. Before the little boy could sense the imminent separation, the Rani had jumped on her horse's back, commanding her men to attack the enemies.

Smith was very cautious; he had hidden a few of his platoons in the eastern and southern ravines. The Rani attacked the British fiercely while her cannons continued to attack General Smith's army. The assault forced Smith to order the Rajput army to destroy the deadly cannons. The Rajput hussars kept falling but marched ahead till they captured the cannons; they were surprised to see women loading the cannons. Without showing a trace of mercy, the Rajputs slaughtered all of them.

The moment the Rani's cannons fell silent, Smith came out with his hiding platoons and attacked her from both sides. She sent a messenger seeking help from the reserve forces of Gwalior. But by that time, Gwalior's army had already surrendered before the British.

The Rani and her handful of soldiers were now stuck between the British bayonets and cannons. Seeing death in their eyes, the Rani's soldiers exhibited audacious valour. The Rani herself was fighting with swords in both hands with the rein of her horse between her teeth. She was making her way out towards the Sonrekha brook while with every passing second, the Rajputs under Smith were inching closer to her.

With swords in both hands, the Rani kept slaughtering the enemy force. When the sun was about to set, one British soldier's bayonet pierced the Queen's back. She retaliated and in a flash, her sword separated the soldier's head from his body.

The badly injured Rani reached a stream but her horse refused to move ahead. The British troops had again trapped her. The eminent threat to her life did not kill her warrior spirit and she kept fighting.

Finally, a British rider came from the back and waved his sword slicing the back of the Rani's head and her right eye. A loyal rider of the Rani's caught her falling body and ran away.

'"Mera Jhansi nahi doongi." She had made that promise.' John Lang remembered their meeting in the palace. 'Kalpi being very formidable, intersected by labyrinths of ravines, impossible for artillery and cavalry to pierce through, was the only place where she could have gone.'

'Sahib, she won the mighty fort of Gwalior and was about to launch the offensive. But, Scindia betrayed her. He was always loyal to the British but pretended sympathy to the Queen as a way of detaining the large body of her troops based in Gwalior,' Badaru was now crying.

'Yes. Badaru, if only Gwalior would help her,' Lang lamented. 'Indeed, she was the only man among the rebels.'

Bibliography

Books

Choudhury, S.B. (1985) 'The Great Revolt', in K.K. Datta and V.A. Narain (eds) *A Comprehensive History of India*, Vol. 11, People's Publishing House, New Delhi.

Dharma Raja, M.K. (2004) *Abbakka Devi: Warrior Queen of Karnataka*, India Perspectives, Bangalore.

Dutt, G.M. and Roy, S. (1988) 'Chennamma of Keladi: The Queen Who Defied Aurangzeb', in Anant Pai (ed) *Amar Chitra Katha*, Amar Chitra Katha Pvt. Ltd, Mumbai.

Eraly, A. (2000) *Emperors of the Peacock Throne*, Penguin Books, New Delhi.

———. (2015) *The Age of Wrath: A History of the Delhi Sultanate*, Penguin Books, New Delhi.

———. (2015) *The Last Spring: Life in India's Last Golden Age, Part II*, Penguin Books, New Delhi.

———. (2015) *The Last Spring: The Saga of the Great Mughals, Part I*, Penguin Books, New Delhi.

Gribble, J.D.B. (1896) *A History of the Deccan*, Luzac & Co., London.

Grover, B.L., Yashpal (1995) *Adhunik Bharat ka Itihas*, S. Chand & Co. Pvt. Ltd., Delhi.

Kaur, Manmohan (1985) *Women in India's Freedom Struggle*, Sterling Publishers Private Limited, New Delhi.

Keay, J. (2000) *India*, Harper Press, London.

Lang J. (2015) *In the Court of the Ranee of Jhansi and Other Travels in*

India, Speaking Tiger, New Delhi.

Malleson, G.B. (1998) *The Indian Mutiny of 1857*, Rupa Publications India Pvt. Ltd, New Delhi.

Mewaram (2014) *Sultan Raziya*, Bhartiya Jnanpith, New Delhi.

Mishra, S. (2010) '1857 ki Veerangana Rani Avantibai', in Badrinarayan, R. Chaudhary and S. Nath (eds) *1857 ka Mahasangram: Vaikalpik Itihas ki Or*, Adhar Prakashan, Panchkula.

Muthanna, I.M. (1977) *Karnataka: History, Administration & Culture*, Lotus Printers, Bangalore.

Patel, T. and Waeerkar, R. (1974) 'Chand Bibi: The Fearless Queen', in Anant Pai (ed) *Amar Chitra Katha*, Amar Chitra Katha Pvt. Ltd, Mumbai.

Prabhupada, Swami A.C.B. (1986) *Bhagwat Gita as It Is*, 2nd ed, The Bhakti Vedanta Book Trust, Mumbai.

Rag, P. (2008) '1857: Vaikalpik Sroton ki Aavshyakata', in Devendra Chaube, Badrinarayan and Hitendra Patel (eds) *1857: Bharat Ka Pahla Mukti Sangharsh*, Praksashan Sansthan, New Delhi.

Raghavan, R., Chavan, H.S. and Kadam, D. (1978) 'The Rani of Kittur: The Defiant Queen', in Anant Pai (ed) *Amar Chitra Katha*, Amar Chitra Katha Pvt. Ltd, Mumbai.

Sahai, M. (1983) 'Dilli Sultanate ki Sthapana', in H. Verma (ed) *Madhyakaleen Bharat: Khand 1*, Delhi University, Delhi.

Sastri, K.A. Nilakanta (1999) *A History of South India*, 4th ed., Oxford University Press, New Delhi.

Sen, S.S. (1999) *Ancient Indian History and Civilisation*, 2nd ed, New Age International Publishers, New Delhi.

Shyam, Radhey (1966) *The Kingdom of Ahmadnagar*, Motilal Banarsidas, Delhi.

Singh, M. and Joshi, H. (1974) 'Abbakka: The Flame of Freedom', in Anant Pai (ed) *Amar Chitra Katha*, Amar Chitra Katha Pvt. Ltd, Mumbai.

———. (1974) 'Rani of Jhansi: The Flame of Freedom', in Anant Pai (ed) *Amar Chitra Katha*, Amar Chitra Katha Pvt. Ltd, Mumbai.

Venkataramanayya, N. and Somasekhara Sarma, M. (1960) 'The

Kakatiyas of Warangal', in G. Yazdani (ed) *The Early History of the Deccan*, Parts VII to XI, Oxford University Press, London.
Verma, V.L. (2014) *Jhansi ki Rani*, Prabhat Prakashan, New Delhi.
———. (2014) *Maharani Durgavati*, Prabhat Prakashan, New Delhi.
Waeerkar, R. (1976) 'Sultana Razia: Empress of India', in Anant Pai (ed) *Amar Chitra Katha*, Amar Chitra Katha Pvt. Ltd, Mumbai.

Internet Resources

Rudramba

1. *Rani Rudrama Devi of Kakatiya Dynasty*, http://mudiraja.weebly.com/05-rani-rudrama-devi-of-kakatiya-dynasty.html accessed on 28 September 2015.

Chand Bibi

2. *Philip Meadows Taylor*, https://en.wikipedia.org/wiki/Philip_Meadows_Taylor accessed on 27 September 2015.

Abbakka

3. *Abbakka Chowta*, https://en.wikipedia.org/wiki/Abbakka_Chowta accessed on 12 August 2015.
4. *Abbakka Rani: the Warrior Queen who defeated the Portuguese*, http://www.hindujagruti.org/articles/85.html accessed on 12 August 2015.
5. Hebbar, N.H. (2005) *The Intrepid Queen: Rani Abbakka Devi of Ullal*, http://www.boloji.com/index.cfm?md=Content&sd=Articles&ArticleID=747 accessed on 12 August 2015.
6. *John III of Portugal*, https://en.wikipedia.org/wiki/John_III_of_Portugal accessed on 11 August 2015.
7. Mishra, K.K. (2002) *Abbakka Rani: the Unsung Warrior Queen*, http://ignca.nic.in/nl001903.htm accessed on 12 August 2015.
8. *Persian-Portuguese War*, https://en.wikipedia.org/wiki/Persian%E2%80%93Portuguese_war accessed on 11 August 2015.
9. *Rani Abbakka: A Bunt Jain Queen*, http://mudiraja.weebly.com/04-rani-abbakka-devi-chowta—a-bunt-jain-queen.html

accessed on 12 August 2015.

10. *Shah Abbas I*, https://en.wikipedia.org/wiki/Abbas_I_of_Persia accessed on 10 August 2015.

Chennamma of Keladi

11. *Keladi Chennamma,* http://yousigma.com/biographies/keladichennamma.html accessed on 13 September 2015.
12. *Rani Chennamma of Keladi* (2008) http://hinduhistory.blogspot.in/2008/02/rani-chennamma-of-keladi.html accessed on 13 September 2015.
13. *Rani Keladi Chennamma of Kelady Dynasty*, http://mudiraja.weebly.com/06-rani-keladi-chennamma-of-kelady-dynasty.html accessed on 12 September 2015.

Tara Bai

14. *Hambirao Mohite,* https://en.wikipedia.org/wiki/Hambirao_Mohite accessed on 16 July 2015.
15. *Sambhaji,* https://en.wikipedia.org/wiki/Sambhaji accessed on 12 July 2015.
16. *Tarabai,* https://en.wikipedia.org/wiki/Tarabai accessed on 21 August 2015.
17. *Third Battle of Panipat,* https://en.wikipedia.org/wiki/Third_Battle_of_Panipat accessed on 18 July 2015.

Chennamma of Kittur

18. *Kittur Chennamma,* https://en.wikipedia.org/wiki/Kittur_Chennamma accessed on 15 August 2015.
19. *Kittur Rani Chennamma: Earliest Ruler to fight British Rule,* http://www.hindujagruti.org/articles/51_kittur-rani-chennamma.html accessed on 15 August 2015.
20. *Kittur Rani Chennamma: the first ever Valiant Queen to fight against the British,* https://hindusoldier.wordpress.com/2013/02/21/kittur-rani-chennamma-the-first-ever-valiant-queen-to-fight-against-the-british/ accessed on 15 August 2015.
21. *Rani Chennamma,* http://www.hinduhistory.info/rani-chennamma/ accessed on 15 August 2015.

Avantibai

22 Bhati, S. and Singh M. (2013) '*1857 ke Swantrata Sangram mein Avantibai ki Bhumika*' in Janitihas (blog), *http://janitihas.blogspot.in/2013/02/1857-avanti-bai-lodhi_19.html* accessed on 28 September 2015.

23. *Rani Avantibai*, http://arisebharat.com/2014/03/20/rani-avantibai/ accessed on 25 September 2015.

Acknowledgements

As always, my wife Dr Adita and our children, Ilina and Agastya, supported me with their encouragement and interest as I narrated these tales to them. I am very grateful.

I am also grateful to my friends Rakesh Tyagi and Rajesh Bhargavji.

My special thanks to Shreya Mukherjee and Shreya Chakraborti, my editors at Rupa Publications, for their encouragement and support.

Made in United States
Cleveland, OH
26 October 2026

46956063R10103